REPRODUCTIVE RITUALS

By the same author

Birth Control in Nineteenth-Century England

Sexuality and Social Order: The debate over the fertility of workers and women in France, 1770–1920

REPRODUCTIVE RITUALS:

The perception of fertility in England from the sixteenth century to the nineteenth century

ANGUS McLAREN

Methuen
London and New York

First published in 1984 by
Methuen & Co. Ltd
11 New Fetter Lane, London EC4P 4EE

Published in the USA by
Methuen & Co.
in association with Methuen, Inc.
733 Third Avenue, New York, NY 10017

Typeset in Great Britain by Keyset Composition,
Colchester, Essex
Printed in Great Britain by Richard Clay,
The Chaucer Press

British Library Cataloguing in Publication Data
McLaren, Angus
Reproductive rituals.
1. Fertility, Human – Great Britain – History
I. Title
304.6'32'0941   HB993

ISBN 0-416-37450-6
ISBN 0-416-37460-3 Pbk

Library of Congress Cataloging in Publication Data
McLaren, Angus.
Reproductive rituals.

Bibliography: p.
Includes index.
1. Fertility, Human – England – History.
2. Fertility, Human – England – Folklore – History.
3. Birth control – England – History.
4. Birth control – England – Folklore – History.
5. Conception – Folklore.   I. Title.
GT2465.G7M35 1984   392'.6   84-1068
ISBN 0-416-37450-6
ISBN 0-416-37460-3 (pbk.)

Contents

In memory of my mother

Acknowledgements

I would like to thank the following for their comments and suggestions: Donna Andrew, John Beattie, Morris Berman, Georgina Born, Jeanne Cannizio, Roger Cooter, Catherine Crawford, John Gillis, Ruth Harris, Ralph Houlbrouke, John Hutchinson, Marlene Legates, David Levine and Geoffrey Quaife. Brian Dippie read the entire manuscript and provided once again both pertinent and preposterous criticisms. Parts of this study were read and useful suggestions for changes were received, at the 1982 Anglo-American Conference of Historians and the 1983 Hunter Symposium at the Wellcome Institute for the History of Medicine. Arlene Tigar McLaren, in the process of finishing her own book, has not had the time to read the manuscript in its entirety but without her proddings it would never have been undertaken. I was able to carry out the work on this study as a result of Faculty Research Grants from the University of Victoria and grants from the Social Sciences and Humanities Research Council of Canada, for which I am greatly appreciative. Enormous help was offered me by the staffs of the Library of the Wellcome Institute for the History of Medicine, the Woodward Medical Library at the University of British Columbia, the British Library, and the Library of the London School of Economics. Some of the material contained in this book first appeared in a different form in the first chapter of my *Birth Control in Nineteenth-Century England* (London: Croom Helm, 1978) and in an article in the *Journal of Sex Research*; I wish to thank the publishers for permission to reprint material from these volumes. Finally, I wish to acknowledge the indispensable aid of those who typed various versions of the manuscript – Vicky Barath, June Belton, Barbara Butler, Dinah Dickie and Gloria Orr.

Introduction:
History and cultural anthropology

This study was sparked by comparing what historians and cultural anthropologists had to say about pre-industrial societies' interest in and ability to control reproduction. Since the nineteenth century anthropologists have devoted a great deal of attention to the study of sexual systems and sexual cultures but it has only been since the late 1960s that historians have seriously investigated family life in early modern Britain and Europe. Edward Shorter stated in 1975 that earlier generations lived in the 'bad old days' when fertility was untrammelled and high birth rates only kept in check by high death rates.[1] David Hunt asserted that women were the passive victims of this tragedy. 'I would conclude that the woman in the old regime exerted no effective control over her own reproductive functions. She conceived, nurtured children, and conceived again according to a rhythm which in origin was biological, and in practice closely related to the whim of her husband.'[2] A similar line has been taken by some demographic historians. John Knodel and Etienne van de Walle have demonstrated that only in the nineteenth century were birth rates brought down, which 'leads us to conclude that family limitation was not a form of behaviour known to the majority prior to the fertility transition and thus not a real option for couples'.[3]

The picture of the pathetic rural mother, the victim of her own fecundity, is painted by both an anti-feminist like Edward Shorter and a feminist like Laurel Thatcher Ulrich.[4] Both E. P. Thompson and Lawrence Stone have stated that poor couples in the early modern period would not think of trying to limit family size. 'The high rate of infant mortality', declares

1

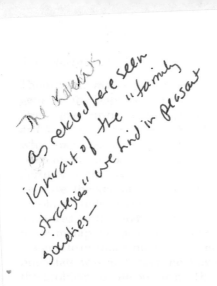

The ... as rebbd here seen / ignorant of the "family strategies" we find in peasant societies —

mily planning; in
notation of time'.[5]
y *The Family, Sex*,
ns up the reasons
hteenth century,
nen and women.
place, he asserts,
the constraints of
equired scientific
rgues, to under-
of reason and so
sive acceptance of
best response to
h control became
ly and morally
acceptable . . . to make planned choices rather than trust to the will of God'. The second reason given by Stone why fertility control was not practised in earlier times was that the pervasive misery of the masses made such foresight pointless. It would require, he states, an actual improvement in the standard of living to make the idea of limiting births meaningful. If a working-class family was impoverished whether it had two or twelve children what difference could birth control make? But 'once there was hope of escape from unpredictable catastrophe it became possible and reasonable to assert one's right to determine and plan one's own future'.[6]

Thus there have been various pessimistic views of family life between 1500 and 1800, describing a society in which, because of the numbing effects of poverty, ignorance and superstition, fertility raged uncontrolled.[7] But it is interesting to compare these views of the reproductive attitudes of pre-industrial England with those of pre-industrial but current cultures. In some peasant cultures, anthropologists tell us, fertility is never found to be 'natural'. Conception, pregnancy, childbirth and nursing are all sociologically determined.[8] 'There is not one single instance on record', asserted Malinowski, 'of a primitive culture in which the process of gestation is left to nature alone'.[9] Anthropologists have uncovered, in pre-industrial societies, a vast range of rules, regulations, taboos, charms and herbal remedies for the purpose of effecting the processes of conception and gestation. The obvious question is, therefore, if 'primitives' around the world could be detected by anthropologists attempting and succeeding in the control of their fertility, why have the same processes not been discovered in pre-industrial England?

This study was carried out because more and more evidence indicated that what cultural anthropologists have revealed about sexual systems in other cultures, could be employed to allow a fruitful re-examination of attitudes towards procreation in early modern England. By observing how anthropologists approached the issue of fertility control it is possible to discover questions that can be asked about the behaviour of earlier generations of English people.[10]

In what ways do anthropologists suggest alternative approaches to the history of fertility control? Their first premise is that only an intimate view of the issues of conception and birth will reveal the role played by cultural concerns in family strategies. A demographic approach that works with large samples, samples usually divorced from their social reality, will not detect differences in motivation.[11] The control of births is part of a total cultural pattern by which a society seeks to regulate its numbers; if the issue is isolated from its social context its reality is lost. For example, when considering the large number of births experienced by English women in earlier times historians have tended to conclude that high fertility indicates lack of fertility control. However, anthropologists' studies indicate that the two are not mutually exclusive. A society's high fertility does not necessarily mean the absence either of the knowledge of control or of a desire to control. In some cultures in which stigmas are attached to barrenness and children are highly valued in economic and cultural terms a high birth rate is sought and large families taken as a demonstration of the community's ability to *control*, by promoting, births. On the other hand other societies may be convinced that their high levels of natality could be even higher if constraints currently employed were not in place. In this case we have an example of high but *limited* birth rates.[12] It is a fact that fertility levels in few societies ever approach their possible biological maxima. Nor are all the communities investigated by anthropologists marked by large families. It would be misleading to retain the view, held by some historians, that in the past extremely high birth and death rates everywhere kept the masses at a subsistence level. But anthropologists have revealed that high fertility rates are not necessarily inherent to pre-industrial societies and they point, as examples, to the Inuit, the Tibetans and the Kaligari bush people.[13]

Both high and low birth rates are used by anthropologists to demonstrate that there is no such thing as 'natural fertility'. 'Natural fertility' has been defined by historians of early modern Europe as untrammelled by contraceptive measures, and fertility within stable sexual unions in the absence of deliberate family size limitation. It was both the theoretical and empirical work of Louis Henry that made it a standard concept in the field of demography. In his first article on the subject in 1953 Henry defined natural fertility as 'fertility of a human population that makes no deliberate efforts to limit births'. He later refined the concept to refer to fertility in the absence of parity-dependent birth control, or 'fertility in the absence of behavior to control births which is . . . bound to the number of children already born and is modified when the number reaches the maximum which the couple does not want to exceed'.[14] Henry recognized that there were populations whose behaviour might affect the level of fertility through prolonging the interval between births while remaining indifferent to the number eventually born. Such behaviour could include breast-feeding, post-natal abstinence and temporary migration separating spouses. But rules affecting the number married, age of marriage, divorce, dowries, residence and sleeping patterns, diet, suckling and so on were obviously crucial. It is thus possible to locate fertility control as a basic adaptive element within the sexual system of a society.

Restrictions on marriage naturally limited the number of births, and the level of nuptiality in early modern England was a key determinant of the level of fertility. Indeed, it has been argued by historical demographers that pre-industrial west European societies (of which England might be seen as the supreme/archetypal case) differed considerably from many Asiatic and African societies in the degree to which attempts to limit fertility within marriage were actively pursued. Lesthaeghe distinguishes between the three processes of 'starting', 'spacing' and 'stopping' in the matter of fertility and stresses the particularly important role for 'starting' the limitation of births by postponing marriage in western Europe.[15] There does seem to be a fairly consistent relationship in the demographic literature suggesting that the late age of marriage and lower proportions ever marrying in Europe were

4

found to coexist with generally high levels of marital fertility.

But it would be a mistake to assume that the level of nuptiality in early modern England was the only determinant of the level of fertility, or that once a woman married her career as childbearer was irrevocably begun and would continue until menopause; or to imply that fertility control that was either volitional or based on any understanding of physiology was impossible. According to the recent biographer of Malthus it was only in the nineteenth century with the manufacture of rubber contraceptives that effective contraception for the married was made possible.[16] Such statements lose credibility when placed in a cross-cultural context. Why should the English have had to wait for manufactured contraceptives when anthropologists have found that primitive peoples have employed a wide range of methods to control fertility – the abstinence of the Yoruba, the post-partum taboos of the Dahomeans and Mossi, the extended nursings of the Ibo, the coitus interruptus of the Tikopia and Bemba, the abortion of the Chagga and Fang, and the douches, suppositories, herbal potions and magical charms of a host of other cultures?[17]

Some methods have been noted. The use of magic to influence fertility has drawn the amused attention of historians from Himes to Shorter as proof of the lack of contraceptive knowledge in earlier periods.[18] For the over-rational historian the magical contraceptive is the ineffective contraceptive. In so judging the issue the historian may not only overlook the possible psychological effects of such charms but also assume that they imply the user's ignorance of basic physiology. Such assumptions are rarely warranted.[19] Anthropologists alert us to the fact that the use of charms along with other fertility-controlling strategies does not indicate simplemindedness. On the contrary, it suggests a complex view of conception in which both the physical and the spiritual are involved. Keith Thomas, in his examination of witchcraft in England, similarly pointed out that in earlier times magic and medicine faded one into the other.[20] The historian of sexuality should accordingly be aware of how anachronistic one can be in using twentieth-century criteria to judge whether or not past contraceptive practices 'worked'.

Abortion also deserves particular attention inasmuch as the history of the practice in England has not been written, yet anthropologists have discovered its employment in every culture they have examined.[21] Historians of early modern England have paid little attention to the issue presumably because they have assumed that its danger to the mother's health and its immorality would have made the practice un-thinkable to most. Anthropologists suggest, however, that the practice can also have some unexpected advantages. In economic terms abortion has the advantage of allowing an individual living in a society near the subsistence level to postpone the issue of controlling pregnancy to a later point in the reproductive cycle so that the calculation of whether or not another child can be supported can be most easily judged.[22] In sexual terms, abortion has the advantage of keeping fertility control within the woman's power: it is simpler than mech-anical contraception; it does not require the co-operation of the male; it does not take place during intercourse; it is under a woman's control. Morokvasic reports that in Yugoslavia where women are very proud of their sexual drive, and where their sexuality and capacity to bear children are closely related – as are their social status and maternity – abortion is a surprisingly suitable means of fertility control:

> Abortion remains virtually the sole fertility control method for Yugoslavs since it leaves open the possibility of having sex and also having the occasional proof of one's virility or fecundity. When a woman has no means other than the maternal role to establish her status, then she may well turn to this even if only potentially. Abortion in this case is almost a symbolic procreation: permitting the capacity to procreate to be tested while ensuring the control of fertility.[23]

Finally, in moral terms, abortion, though condemned by male doctors, lawyers and priests, may be far more acceptable to women than one might first anticipate. Fatima Mernissi, in her study of Moroccan mothers, concluded that women 'are generally not easily impressed or influenced by formal religious or legal codes. Family planning officials apparently make a mistake if they ascribe too much importance to religious and legal authorities in the formation of women's attitudes towards fertility control'.[24] Such reports are very suggestive; a similar, separate female sexual culture in early modern England therefore seems likely.

In highlighting the importance of abortion anthropologists alert us to the fact that men and women might have different means and ends in mind when contemplating fertility control.[25] Those historians who have talked about 'family planning' have tended to assume that the family is a tension-free unit. Anthropologists have been more sensitive to sexual tensions and ask such questions as: who takes the initiative in sexual encounters? Who is supposed to gain more pleasure? Who controls fertility? Can the woman use her control of fertility against the man? Does the man perceive a limitation of the woman's births as a sign of his loss of control over her? By including the woman's concerns in the discussion of fertility control one is led to recognize that limitation of births might be sought – not just by the man because of simple economic concerns as some historians would have us believe – but by the woman to avoid repeated miscarriages, difficult pregnancies, ill health and the resultant suffering subjected on already existing children. Here is another chapter of family history awaiting its chronicler.

In reviewing the reasons why women might seek to control fertility anthropologists make the crucial point that in other cultures it was the timing of births, not their limitation in number, that was often the first priority. Other societies employed a variety of practices that, though they resulted in a diminished fertility, were often turned to for other reasons. Anthropologists point, as examples, to 'bundling' and limited pre-marital sex play that allowed marriages to be postponed until couples were sexually or psychologically mature, religious celibacy, abortion in the case of illegitimate pregnancies, 'eugenic' infanticide and prolonged nursing in order to protect the young child. In the treatment of situations in which couples deliberately attempted to space their children but were unconcerned with – or even opposed to – limiting the ultimate family size, one again raises the troublesome ambiguity of the term 'natural fertility'. Recent research in non-European societies suggests that such situations may be more common than previously recognized. For example, surveys in Nigeria and Indonesia undertaken in areas where post-natal abstinence is common indicate that this practice is explicitly viewed by substantial portions of the population as a deliberate attempt to space births for the benefit of the health of both mother and child. In these cases at least, post-partum abstinence is not simply a 'taboo' practised by couples largely unconscious of its effects on fertility, but rather is viewed by the indigenous

7

population as a deliberate and rational attempt to space births. In both cultures, however, there is little indication that this practice is related to any desire to limit family size. In the western twentieth-century mind birth control primarily means limitation of numbers; in other cultures control over births arose out of a concern of not only how many children were born but of who had them, when, how far apart, and up to what age.[26] The anthropologically informed historian would expect to find the same preoccupations and practices in early modern England, in particular the extension of nursing which had as its purpose the protection of mother and child and as a consequence the wide spacing of births.

A further valuable insight offered by anthropologists that seems applicable to this study relates to the problems that occur when two sexual cultures clash. For historians who assume the dominance of bourgeois values it was undeniably a 'good thing' when the medicalized, commercialized contraceptive knowledge of the middle classes percolated down to the lower orders and usurped their old reliance on magic and herbal potions.[27] A similar scenario is sketched out by anthropologists describing the intrusion of Europeans into non-western societies, but the conclusion is different. They argue that prior to contact native cultures had their own established demographic balance. The effect of the arrival of doctors and missionaries condemning and attempting to replace traditional forms of fertility control was to destroy the old balance.[28] In theory the entry of modern, western scientific ideas should have led to more effective fertility control; in practice the old controls were lost and rapid increase in population ensued because European forms of fertility regulation were long viewed with hostility. The most sophisticated method of birth control does not work if it is not used and it is not used if it violates the traditional views of a society. Thus in Sri Lanka the condom is feared because it is believed to prevent a necessary exchange of blood, and in Morocco and Iran the pill is avoided because it is thought to be poisonous.[29]

Did the same sort of surge in fertility take place in England for similar sorts of reasons at the end of the eighteenth century? Can the doctors who moved into obstetrics and so displaced midwives, and the jurists who made women's recourse to abortion a statutory offence in 1803 be usefully compared to the missionaries in Africa who in the next century 'campaigned vigorously against a number of measures by which women controlled their fertility, including the segregation of the sexes after childbirth, the whole practice of polygamy, and women's secret societies used for, among other things, initiation in traditional methods of fertility control'?[30]

A population revolution did occur in England between 1750 and 1850, but until recently the great increase in numbers was attributed to a fall in the death rate, not to any surge in the birth rate. The argument ran that fertility was consistently high through the seventeenth and eighteenth centuries.[31] A more recent account – E. A. Wrigley and R. S. Schofield's *The Population History of England, 1541–1871* – has overthrown the old interpretation and re-emphasized the role of fertility. Wrigley and Schofield found that in fact fertility fell in the seventeenth century from its sixteenth-century level. The gross reproduction rate in the 1500s of 2.8 declined to 1.9 by 1650, swung back to 2.3 in 1756 and only climbed to 3.06 in 1816. As a result, England's population of 5.058 million in 1701 was actually smaller than the 5.092 million of 1641. It was between 1741 and 1801 when the old constraints on fertility were loosened that the population surged from 5.576 to 8.664 million. Wrigley and Schofield attribute these eighteenth-century gains in fertility primarily to a reduction in the age of marriage.[32] Wrigley argued in an earlier article, however, that when explaining ultimate family size the employment or non-employment of birth control techniques had also to be taken into account. David Levine, Keith Wrightson and Daniel Scott Smith have advanced evidence which indicates that age of marriage was not the sole regulator of fertility.[33] M. W. Flinn has likewise argued that detailed research into the demographic statistics of seventeenth- and eighteenth-century England reveals a significant drop in the age of the mother at the time of the birth of her last child – a positive sign of the employment of fertility-controlling strategies.[34] In short, quantifiers now agree that fertility was variable in early modern England and not wholly biologically determined.

There are two other crucial revisions of the older interpretations of English family history. First, the reappraisal of the notion that 'romantic love' did not exist prior to the 1700s. A pessimistic view of male/female relationships in the early modern period was popularized both by Shorter and Stone. According to Shorter, men viewed their spouses with

9

calculated indifference, remained emotionally distant and based their marital strategies on their preoccupations with property considerations.[35] Stone argued that such cold relationships only began to give way to affectionate 'companionate marriages' in the late seventeenth and early eighteenth centuries.[36] Keith Wrightson has shown, however, how easy it is, by relying simply on prescriptive literature which doggedly repeats maxims on the necessity of a wife's subservience, to paint an overly black picture of conjugal relations.[37] Wrightson's plea for a more cautious analysis of marriage which would highlight the subtle balance of patriarchal and companionate concerns has been echoed by Michael MacDonald.[38] In his fascinating exploration of the medical case books of a seventeenth-century physician MacDonald has revealed that even in a patriarchal world 'romantic love', with its accompanying seductions and heartbreaks, did exist.

MacDonald's investigations have also turned up evidence of the searing grief seventeenth-century parents experienced at the loss of a child,[39] modifying the assertions that childhood was disparaged in the early modern period and that high infant mortality rates made it psychologically too risky for parents in the sixteenth and seventeenth centuries to pour out their love on offspring.[40] It is an exaggeration to speak of some sudden massive change in parental affection in the eighteenth century: parents in past times were frequently distant and did demand obedience, but at the same time they obviously took pleasure in children for whom they often made immense sacrifices.[41]

It will not be possible in this book to venture down all the avenues of investigation suggested by anthropologists. Nor would such a course be prudent. Natalie Davis has wisely cautioned: 'We consult anthropological writings not for pre-scriptions, but for suggestions; not for universal rules of human behaviour, but for relevant comparisons. There is no substitute for extensive work in the historical sources'.[42] Keeping this admonition in mind, in the chapters that follow an attempt will be made to exploit the more fruitful suggestions of anthropology in analysing the attitudes of early modern English men and women towards conception and pro-creation.[43] The first chapter examines their understanding of the relationship of pleasure and procreation; chapter two, their efforts to promote fertility; chapter three, their reasons for and ways of limiting births; chapter four, their views on abortion.

The final chapter analyses the campaign led by jurists and medical men to intrude on traditional means of fertility control. Cultural anthropology which provides useful insights on how to discover the harmonious workings of a culture is less helpful in grappling with the problem of change. The purpose of this book is to present both the traditional view of procreation and the transformations it underwent; it will employ anthropological suggestions but will remain basically a historical survey.

The great handicap of the historian hoping to apply the anthropologist's insights is that the former's subjects inhabit not only another culture, but other centuries. No friendly informant is at hand to describe and explain the reproductive rituals of early modern England. A good deal of research is required to track down useful information. The most readily available discussions of traditional attitudes towards procreation are those written by doctors who were often hostile to fertility-regulating practices. Accordingly, their accounts have to be treated with some scepticism, particularly when these male, urban professionals claim to be reporting the opinions of female, rural patients. Medical accounts do contain, however, a wealth of information and can be supplemented with almanacs, herbals, folk-songs, proverbs, court reports, literary accounts, letters, diaries and unpublished family receipt books. In exploiting such sources this study does not have the goal of analysing the fertility rate in past centuries, but by using contemporary accounts to reveal the mental structures and sexual vocabularies of past generations in order to discover not only what happened in the process of conception, gestation and birth but what people *thought* happened.

1
The pleasures of procreation:
traditional and biomedical theories of conception

The popular conceptions of female physiology are generally held by women of all social groups in Maragheh, regardless of their educational background. Some educated women (and men) may hold both a modified version of the popular model and a simplified version of the biomedical model. But only the town's physicians appear to dismiss the popular myth *in toto*, in favor of the biomedical model of female physiology.
Mary-Jo Delvecchio Good, 'Of blood and babies: the relationship of popular Islamic physiology to fertility,' *Social Science and Medicine*, 14B (1980), 151.

A recent chronicler of eighteenth-century childbearing has argued that the dangers and diseases which inevitably accompanied parturition were so great that women in past times must have loathed and feared sex.[1] But cultural anthropology's most important insight is that every aspect of social life is culturally conditioned: the ways in which people perceive their experiences are as important as the experiences themselves.[2] To begin our investigations of the patterning of human fertility we will in this chapter seek to understand how English people in the past viewed the process of procreation and how such views began to change in the course of the eighteenth century.

In 1776 the Scottish surgeon John Hunter supervised the first successful attempt at human artificial insemination. Hunter instructed a linen-draper who suffered from hypospadias how to use a warm syringe to impregnate his wife. The operation worked and pregnancy ensued, but because of Hunter's fear of the criticisms of moralists it was only reported posthumously twenty-three years later in the *Philosophical Transactions* of the Royal Society.[3] Hunter's success deserves, perhaps, more attention from historians because no other act so dramatically demonstrated the separation of the principles of sexual pleasure and procreation which is said to have occurred as the 'modern mind' emerged.

How did early modern English men and women perceive sexuality? Was it pleasurable? Was it a similar experience for both sexes? According to the historians who in the 1970s plotted the rise of the modern family, it was only in the eighteenth century that the enjoyment of sexuality became, for women, at least a possibility. Lawrence Stone, Edward Shorter and Randolph Trumbach all advance what is largely a Whig interpretation of the history of the family according to which only relatively recently did love, affection and a concurrent concern for the sexual gratification of one's mate emerge.[4] They attribute the possibility of women's enjoyment of sexuality to the growth of a new individualism linked to market capitalism and to the freedom from pregnancies offered by the expansion of contraceptive knowledge. There is much of value in such arguments concerning the eighteenth century, but they fail to explain why in the nineteenth the double standard continued to hold sway: far from enjoining women to anticipate sexual pleasure, the majority of early Victorian writers who broached the subject counselled stoicism and passivity. Such an interpretation also fails to explain why – if the 'pleasure principle' were only to appear in the eighteenth century – the sixteenth and seventeenth centuries were marked by an earthy attitude towards sexuality strikingly absent in the sentimental late 1700s and the prudish early 1800s.

Hunter's work does provide a useful benchmark against which such shifts in both popular and scientific attitudes towards procreation can be plotted. In this study the literature devoted to the issues of sexual pleasure and procreation prior to Hunter's activities will be reviewed with the intent of casting a fresh light on the history of English attitudes towards sexuality. It will be argued that from the sixteenth to the eighteenth centuries it was commonly assumed that women not only found pleasure in sexual intercourse but that they positively had to if the union were to be a fruitful one. It was only in the 1700s that a new scientific appreciation of the process of procreation began to spread, which held that pleasure and procreation were not necessarily linked. As a consequence, by the beginning of the nineteenth century one could speak of two sexual cultures: a 'low' culture of traditional beliefs in which women's sexuality was accepted, and a 'high' culture of scientific understanding in which women's sexuality had little place.[5] We will be asking the sorts of questions that anthropologists, sensitive to the issue of sexual tensions, have posed – who takes the initiative in sexual encounters? who is supposed to gain more pleasure? who controls fertility? – in an effort to understand why the answers made to such questions in the seventeenth century differed from those of the nineteenth century.

The evidence most often advanced to support the argument that sixteenth- and seventeenth-century attitudes towards sexuality were not 'puritanical' is, ironically enough, drawn primarily from Puritan sources. From Edmund Morgan to Edmund Leites the assertion has been made that Puritans in both England and New England recognized the importance of love, friendship and sexuality in marriage.[6] Traditional Christianity portrayed women as the daughters of Eve and accordingly as lacking in rational control and sexually voracious. A woman's innate interest in sex was considered not so much a matter of her sensibly seeking pleasure as giving in to self-destructive urges. With the rise of the ideal of the 'spiritualized household' in both humanist and Puritan thought in the sixteenth century, however, there came a new legitimation of marital sexuality, a stress on the virtues of family life, and an acceptance of female sexual needs as natural. Women's libidinal drives were taken by Protestants as a good thing inasmuch as they helped hold together the family, whereas conservative Catholics, so the argument runs, continued to prize celibacy and view female sexuality with distaste. The Protestant ethic was echoed by William Gouge in *Of Domesticall Duties* (1622) who claimed spouses owed each other 'due benevolence', and declared 'To deny this duty being justly required, is to deny a due debt, and to give Satan a great advantage'. This Puritan pamphleteer went on to assert that even after a woman was pregnant, sexual relations should continue: 'Conception is not the only end of this duty: for it is to be rendered to such as are barren'.[7] Similarly, Thomas Gataker

15

in *A Good Wife, God's Gift* (1623) claimed, 'In the first place cometh the Wife, as the first and principall blessing, and the Children in the next. . . . If Children bee a Blessing, then the root whence they spring ought much more to bee so esteemed'.[8] In short, such writers shifted the focus on the purpose of marriage from procreation to companionship.

Such interpretations are useful, but a reliance on religious tracts should not overshadow far more obvious sources relating to sexuality: the traditional medical texts.[9] In the large corpus of works devoted to the questions of conception and gestation, sexuality necessarily figured centrally. How one moved from 'non-being' to 'being' was from the time of the Greeks a key philosophical and scientific conundrum. It gave rise to an extended discussion over the centuries of embryological development. It was a discussion which, until the new medical experimentation of the sixteenth century, was highly speculative, one in which laymen, doctors and priests all participated and accepted as given the linking of pleasure and procreation.

Early modern Europeans looked back to Aristotle, Hippocrates and Galen for explanations of how life was created. Aristotle, ignorant of the functions of the ovaries and testicles, believed both male and female produced 'sperma' from their blood – seed from the male and menstrual fluid from the female. The woman because of her natural coldness could not manufacture real seed and as proof Aristotle noted: 'A sign that the female does not emit the kind of seed that the male emits, and that generation is not due to the mixing of both as some hold, is that often the female conceives without experiencing the pleasure that occurs in intercourse'.[10] Given Aristotle's preconceptions regarding male dominance, the male fluid was qualitatively superior; he asserted that it provided the elements of form and movement for the new being, while the female fluid was the source of its matter and passivity. Aristotle suggested that, as in the making of cheese the inert milk was activated by rennet, so too in procreation the active semen produced life from the passive menstrual fluid. He went so far, some have argued, as to deprive women not only of pleasure, but even of maternity and presented them as being little more than incubators. Beyond this, he claimed that semen tried to produce the highest form of life, that is the male; should it fail, the result was an imperfect product, the female.[11]

More popular in the long run than Aristotle's views were

those of Hippocrates who on the whole tended towards an egalitarian model of procreation. He argued that because of the 'intensity of the pleasure involved', the seminal fluids were distillations drawn from all parts of both spouses' bodies and accordingly hereditary traits of either could appear.[12] The two fluids or 'semence' were similar in nature and their mixing produced life. This Hippocratic line was taken up by Galen in the second century AD who attempted to synthesize it with Aristotelian medicine.[13] This compilation of medical theories was to dominate western thought for the next fifteen hundred years. For the purposes of this study, what is of interest is that in contrast to Aristotle's male-oriented explanation of pro-creation the Galenic thesis was 'feminist' inasmuch as both sexes were presented as contributing equally in conception and accordingly both had to experience pleasure. The female seed was said to move like the male and the fact that a woman could not bear children if her ovaries were removed was advanced as proof that she was more than the mere 'nest' Aristotle suggested. Anatomically, the two sexes were presented in Galenic accounts as complementary, the difference being that the man's genitalia were external and the woman's internal. The clitoris was likened to the penis and the ovaries considered 'testicles' or 'stones' that produced seed. The male seed was, it must be said, depicted by Galenists as superior in having 'spiritual' qualities lacking in the female, but Galen's repro-ductive schema was nevertheless far more egalitarian than Aristotle's.

The semence or two-seed theory was to have a long life in western culture.[14] Thomas Raynald asserted that the woman's seed differed from the man's but was no less perfect and her sensual appetites no less demanding:

> For if that the God of nature had not instincted and inset in the body of man and woman such a vehement and ardent appetite and lust, the one lawfully to company with the other, neyther man nor woman would ever have been so attentive to the works of generation and increasement of posterity.[15]

Why, asked Nathaniel Highmore, would women have 'testicles' if not for the purpose of producing seed? 'When also in coition ye shall observe the same delight and concussion as in Males; why should we suppose Nature, beyond her

17

custome, should abound in superfluities and uselesse partes?'[16] Sir Thomas Browne advanced the same views when rebutting the report that a woman could be passively impregnated by bathing in a tub in which a man had left semen. ''Tis a new and unseconded way in history to fornicate at a distance, and much offendeth the rules of physic, which say, there is no generation without joint emission, nor only a virtual, but corporal and carnal contraction'.[17] William Harvey provided a useful summing up of early seventeenth-century views:

> Conception, according to the opinion of medical men, takes place in the following way: during intercourse the male and the female dissolve in one voluptuous sensation, and inject their seminal fluids (geniturae) into the cavity of the uterus, where that which each contributes is mingled with that which the other supplies, the mixture having from both equally the faculty of action and the force of matter; and according to the predominance of this or that geniture does the progeny turn out male or female.[18]

Although the microscope was to permit in the late seventeenth century the beginnings of a more precise definition of the different contributions of the two sexes in procreation, one still found in the popular literature of the late eighteenth century the assumption that the seed of the two were similar. Nicolas Venette spoke of two seeds in *Conjugal Love Reveal'd* (1720), John Maubray in *The Female Physician* (1724) declared that both sexes contributed 'seminal matter', and the best-known of the popular sex manuals, *Aristotle's Masterpiece*, held (until the 1755 edition) to the semence view.[19]

What was the importance of the continuation of the belief that the two sexes both produced seed? In reviewing the literature in 1755 Michel Procope-Couteau noted that to hold such a view implied that both sexes had to experience pleasure in order to procreate.[20] Indeed, in the popular literature, what was most striking was the maintenance of basically Galenic theories of equal responsibility and pleasure in sexual activity.[21] Such texts continued to ask the traditional sorts of questions about conception and gestation: do women experience pleasure? How does conception occur? How can it be prevented or encouraged? Can one predetermine the sex of offspring? The new scientific literature of the late seventeenth century shelved these old questions – at least explicitly – and

18

explored the narrower issues of the organization and development of the embryo. Whether or not the scientific approach was
free of sexual bias is discussed at the end of this chapter but it is
first necessary to provide an account of procreation as
described in the traditional texts.

The best example of the popular works on sexuality was
Aristotle's Masterpiece, the anonymously authored compendium of information that drew from the works of Nicholas
Culpeper, Albertus Magnus and common folklore.[22] The first
editions appeared in the late seventeenth century and in the
eighteenth century there were more editions of it than of any
other medical text. Over time it was viewed by the respectable
as being in increasingly bad taste. In fact, it changed very little
and, if anything, became more modest in its anatomical
descriptions. Attitudes towards it changed, however, because
it crystallized and maintained what were in effect late
seventeenth-century beliefs about sexuality.[23] By drawing on
Aristotle's Masterpiece and other pre-scientific accounts, it is
possible to piece together a picture of early modern sexual
beliefs.

The first point made in such manuals is that women
experience pleasure in the sexual act. According to *Aristotle's
Masterpiece*, at the age of fourteen or fifteen the menses 'incite'
the body and mind of a girl. If the young woman is deprived of
sex she ultimately becomes a 'green and weasel coloured' old
maid. For the married, deprived of companionship by the
death of a spouse, there is the additional problem of stilling a
delicious habit. Such women were described as the 'brisk'
widows whose passions were difficult to calm.[24]

Sexual pleasure was, according to the popular texts, not
simply vaginal. Great attention was paid to the importance of
the clitoris. According to the *Masterpiece* it was clitoral
stimulation that gave 'delights' and such knowledge was
essential 'for without this, the fair sex neither desire mutual
Embraces nor have pleasure in 'em, nor conceive by 'em'.[25]
Henry Bracken in *The Midwife's Companion* (1737) likewise
stated that the clitoris 'by its fullness of nerves and exquisite
sense affords unspeakable Delight'.[26] Sibly wrote in 1794 that
both sexes necessarily experienced 'voluptuous gratification'.[27]
Indeed, the suggestion was made in works like *Conjugal Love
Reveal'd* and *Aristotle's Masterpiece* that women might experience more pleasure than men; that they would be 'more

19

recreated and delighted in the Venerial Act' because they both gave and received seed while men only gave.[28]

The second point made in the texts was that women not only experienced pleasure, they were actively seeking it in sexual embraces. These were certainly not the passive Victorians lying back and thinking of the Empire. Lazarus Riverius in *The Practice of Physick* (1658) poetically imagined that the woman's womb,

> skipping as it were for joy, may meet her Husband's Sperm, graciously and freely receive the same, and draw it into its innermost Cavity or Closet, and withal bedew and sprinkle it with her own Sperm, and powered forth in that pang of Pleasure, that so by the commixture of both, Conception may arise.[29]

James McMath presented the same scene while describing in *The Expert Midwife* (1694) the causes of infertility:

> *Sterility* happens likewise, from the Womans Disgust, and Satiety of the Venereal Embrace; or her dullness and insensibility therein: When the Orifice bids shut against the *Yard*: Which else (while eager upon it, strenuously and naturally *Tickled* and *Roused* therein) applyes to it, delightfully opens, and ravenously attracts the mans *Seed* (which is then sufficiently darted into the Recesses of the *Womb*) emits also her own: Whence *Conception*.[30]

Bracken and Sibly described the womb 'embracing' the penis[31] while Guillemeau declared that

> in some Women the wombe is so greedy, and lickerish that it doth even come down to meet nature, sucking, and (as it were) snatching the same, though it remaine only about the mouth and entrance of the outward orifice thereof.[32]

There could, it was recognized, be problems arising from women's sexual desires. Jane Sharp argued that 'the most frequent cause of Barrenness in young lusty women . . . is . . . their great desire of copulation'.[33]

The third point made in the texts was that the pleasure of the woman was necessary to ensure conception. Venereal delights opened the cervix so admitting the man's seed and precipitating the woman's. Philip Barrough asserted in 1583, 'Also unwilling carnall copulation for the most part is vaine and barren: for love causeth conception, and therefore loving women do conceave often'.[34] Riverius held that it was enjoyment that led the woman to give 'down sufficient quantity of Spirits wherewith her Genitals ought to swel at the instant of Generation'.[35] Nicholas Culpeper stated in *A Directory for Midwives* (1656): 'Want of Love between man and wife, is another cause of Barrenness. That there is an Essential Vital Spirit in the Seed of both sexes, is without all question'.[36] John Sadler agreed:

> Aetuis and Sylvius ascribe one maine cause of barrennesse to compeld copulation, as when parents enforce their daughters to have husbands contrary to their liking, therein marrying their bodies but not their hearts and where there is want of love, there for the most part is no conception; as appears in women which are deflowered against their own will.[37]

Indeed, so widespread was the belief that affection was necessary for conception that it was held that rapes were necessarily sterile. Should a woman who was assaulted bear a child, it could be advanced as proof of her complicity. Samuel Farr in *Elements of Medical Jurisprudence* asserted, 'For without the enjoyment of pleasure in the venereal act no conception can probably take place'.[38]

Any physical problem that rendered the pleasure of the woman difficult to achieve was also believed to hamper procreation. John Pechey referred, for example, to 'some distemper in the Vessels dedicated to generation, and then the woman perceives very little or no pleasure in the act of copulation'.[39] John Bulwer warned, 'circumcision detracts somewhat from the delight of women by lessening their titillation'.[40] Jane Sharp directed particular attention to the clitoris in *The Compleat Midwife's Companion* (1725). It was the clitoris, in her words, which 'makes Women lustful and take delight in Copulation; and were it not for this they would have no desire nor delight, nor would they ever conceive'.[41]

The variety of sources one can draw on to illustrate the continued vitality of Galenic ideas provides support for one of the main contentions of this study – that until the seventeenth century there existed in England a common culture of procreational knowledge in which women's sexual pleasure was seen both by laymen and doctors as necessary for fecundity. In the seventeenth century this common culture was undermined.

What one finds is that a new 'high' culture of scientific embryology emerged that severed the traditional linking of pleasure and procreation: what had been the common culture became the 'low' culture. As indicated by the reprintings of traditional works such as *Aristotle's Masterpiece*, the older interpretations did not disappear, but they were increasingly viewed by the educated and respectable as aspects of the mind of the lewd and vulgar.

From the late sixteenth century onwards, medical scientists who adopted the experimental method were faced with the problem of reconciling their new observations with the models of procreation set out by Aristotle, Hippocrates and Galen. The first discoveries were incorporated in the old model, but as contradictory evidence accumulated it became necessary to construct a new paradigm.[42] The dominant view of embryological development up until the sixteenth century has been called epigenetic, that is, that all parts of the new creation developed simultaneously. The weakness of the theory was that it did not satisfactorily explain how such a complicated process as the creation of life took place. A rival theory to that of epigenesis was that of preformation. Some early writers like Plato and Aeschylus argued that a miniature embryonic life was already in place within the parent – like an egg – and embryological development only consisted of growth, not creation.[43] Such an argument allowed one to avoid the issue of how life was created, but the problem it encountered was that no human egg had been discovered. William Harvey has been hailed by some as the founder of modern embryology for his 1651 work, *De generatione animalium*, but in fact he did not find an egg and he also failed to find semen in the uterus and so fell back on a contagion theory to explain conception. He followed an epigenetic line of reasoning and held that the egg was the *product*, not the cause, of conception.[44]

The real changes in embryological thought came with the emergence of preformation theories in the late seventeenth and early eighteenth centuries. On the continent, Malpighi's important work on the embryological development of the chick provided the basis for a more sophisticated view of conception.

> By its very nature the uterus is a field for growing the seeds, that is to say the ova, sown upon it. Here the eggs are fostered, and here the parts of the living [foetus], when they

have further unfolded, become manifest and are made strong. Yet although it has been cast off by the mother and sown, the egg is weak and powerless and so requires the energy of the semen of the male to initiate growth.[45]

In England, Henry Power and William Croone have been credited with advancing similar preformation theories in the 1660s but the breakthrough came when Renier de Graaf, without the aid of the microscope, discovered what were to be known as the Graafian follicles that contained the mammalian egg.[46] De Graaf's work was available in England by 1672. In fact, the mammalian egg itself was not found until 1827 by von Baer, but the view that the woman, like the chicken, held within her miniature offspring, gained rapid popularity in the scientific community.[47] Thus in John Case's *The Angelical Guide* (1697) are references to the human egg being shaken by the sperm into the fallopian tubes; Joseph Blondel went so far as to refer to semen as mere manure for the ovum; Alexander Hamilton in 1781 declared that the child existed in the ovaries and the act of generation was 'only the means intended by providence to supply it with life'; and William Cullen's edition of Albertus Haller while reviewing conflicting theories on generation held that the foetus was only excited into life by the 'seminal worms'.[48]

The preformationist school contained two separate groups: the ovists – those who held that the miniature being already existed in the mother's egg – and the animalculists – those who argued that a tiny being existed in the spermatozoa. The strength of the ovist argument was based on the analogy with egg-laying animals; the animalculists, on the other hand, singled out the discovery by Leeuwenhoek in 1677 of microscopic beings in semen. The animalculists either denied the existence of the egg or argued that it only existed to provide nourishment for the tiny beings within the drop of semen. As in Aristotle's original formulation the woman was again perceived as little more than a nest or 'nidus'.

Whatever the preferred line of attack, preformation theories budded in the 1670s and blossomed in the first half of the eighteenth century.[49] They presented an image of a mono-parental embryo in which conception implied simply an enlargement of what was already there.[50] There was no 'creation' *per se*. The power of this new theory was based in part on microscopic findings. Indeed the microscope, in revealing a miniature hidden world, fired men's imaginations with the idea of worlds even tinier. The theory was also supported by ideological concerns. It nicely countered the radically rationalist view of the Cartesians that the law of motion had in the beginning created life which in turn supported the concept of abiogenesis or spontaneous generation. The idea of pre-existence or *emboîtement* also complemented seventeenth-century Calvinist and Jansenist ideas of predestination. Science could be seen as confirming the religious idea that all men had been created by God at one point in time.[51] For example, Swammerdam noted that in embryology

> even the foundation of original sin itself would already have been discovered, since the whole of mankind would have been concealed in the loins of Adam and Eve, and to this could be added as a necessary consequence that when these eggs have been exhausted the end of mankind will be at hand.[52]

John Wilkins agreed that the microscope proved the existence of some 'wise intelligent being' and William Paley exulted in the fact that the scientific investigation of reproduction made it more, rather than less, mysterious: 'He [the parent] is in total ignorance why that which is produced took its present form rather than any other. It is for him only to be astonished by the effect'.[53] Science could thus be turned to defend Christianity against mechanical, rationalist arguments.

The pre-existence and preformation theories were not without their weaknesses. How did one explain hereditary traits that might vary from child to child, and the polyp's ability (discovered in the 1740s) to regenerate itself? And on a common-sense level, was one really to believe that Adam and Eve contained within them every generation of mankind ever to live?[54] Clearly this was a theory that easily lent itself to spoofing, a temptation given in to by writers like Sterne.[55] Moreover, the defenders of the animalculist theory had the particular problem of explaining why, if each sperm was a potential man, God permitted the wholesale slaughter of millions of beings in every sexual act.

For present purposes what is most interesting is how the theories related to the role of the sexes. One finds that the animalculists presented women as being little more than passive recipients of the male gift and returned them to their Aristotelian role of breeding-machines. The ovist line of argument would appear at first glance to have been more 'feminist' inasmuch as it credited the mother with carrying preformed beings. In fact the ovists also portrayed the woman as playing a role that was far more passive than that attributed to her by the defenders of the old semence or two-seed theory which had argued that the woman had to be aroused and delighted for conception to occur. The ovists' belief was that her active involvement was minimal: the sperm was active and the egg almost inert. The egg was presented by scientists as 'shaken' into life by the sperm or allowed by its intervention to 'escape' into the fallopian tube. William Smellie, for example, wrote:

> The *Ovum* being impregnated, is squeezed from its *Nidus* or husk into the tube by the contraction of the *Fimbria*, and thus disengaged from its attachments to the *Ovarium*, is endowed with a circulating force by the *Animalculum*, which has a *vis vitae* in itself.[56]

In the latter half of the eighteenth century the inherent weaknesses of the preformation theory resulted in a re-awakened interest in epigenetic views. But there was not a return to the theory of the double semence concept of two homogeneous fluids – rather one saw the elaboration of the idea of two distinct sorts of building blocks for the new creation.[57] For the purposes of this study what is important to note is that in stressing the idea of different male and female sex roles both preformation theories and the later, more sophisticated epigenetic theories undercut the older notion of the necessity of both men and women experiencing sexual pleasure.

The common argument advanced in histories of science is that between the sixteenth and nineteenth centuries scholasticism slowly but surely gave way to empiricism.[58] Nonetheless as embryological thought developed, although the emerging science was in detail more accurate than Galen's ideas – for example, in demonstrating the differentiation of functions in male and female sexual organs – it did not give rise to a more satisfactory general explanation of procreation than that sketched out two thousand years before. Indeed, the new explanation appeared in many ways impoverished inasmuch as it said less and less about the social and cultural aspects of

25

sexuality that ordinary men and women assumed were of utmost importance.

Women's pleasure in sexuality had been traditionally justified on the grounds that their sexual organs were very much like men's. Men had to be aroused to ejaculate and it followed logically enough that women also had to experience pleasure if they were to produce seed. Modern science removed this myth by demonstrating that men and women were anatomically different, and that the ovaries were not 'testicles' producing seed. This new knowledge enabled John Hunter to direct the first successful attempt at human artificial insemination. Theoretically, there was no reason why such more accurate and detailed accounts of physiology should have led to a denigration of women's rights to pleasure, but in practice they did.[59]

The new embryological knowledge of the sperm and the egg – the one active and the other purportedly passive – led to new expectations, or was employed to rationalize new expectations, of differing male and female sexual experiences. William Harvey began this reappraisal of sexual performance innocently enough when he observed that not all females presented an 'effusion of fluid' during intercourse:

> But passing over the fact that the females of all the lower animals, and all women do not experience any such emission of fluid, and that conception is nowise impossible in cases where it does not take place, for I have known several, who without anything of the kind were sufficiently prolific, and even some who after experiencing such an emission and having had great enjoyment, nevertheless appeared to have lost somewhat of their wonted fecundity; and then an infinite number of instances might be quoted of women, who, although they have great satisfaction in intercourse, still emit nothing, and yet conceive.[60]

But those who followed Harvey chose to stress the notion that the pleasure of women was not only unnecessary for procreation but was probably not even attainable. De la Vauguion observed in 1699, 'We see every day, that some women are impregnated without emission of Seed, or receiving the least Pleasure'.[61] Procope-Couteau asked in 1755 if it were not true that many women never felt pleasure during the sexual act.[62] An anonymous author writing in 1789 asserted that pleasure

26

was felt by few women but was in any event not necessary.[63] Fodéré informed his women patients that in place of passion 'complaisance, tranquillity, silence, and secrecy are necessary for a prolific coition'.[64] By the mid-nineteenth century Dr Acton was declaring:

> there can be no doubt that sexual feeling in the female is in the majority of cases in abeyance . . . and even if raised (which in many instances it never can be) is very moderate compared with that of the male. . . . As a general rule, a modest woman seldom desires any sexual gratification for herself. She submits to her husband, but only to please him and, but for the desire of maternity, would far rather be relieved from his attentions.[65]

Patients, however, did not appear to abandon old theories as quickly as their doctors. In the 1860s Sims complained that it was still

> the vulgar opinion, and the opinion of many savants that, to ensure conception, sexual intercourse should be performed with a certain degree of completeness, that would give an exhaustive satisfaction to both parties at the same moment. How often do we hear husbands complain of coldness on the part of the wives; and attribute to this the failure to procreate. And sometimes wives are disposed to think, though they never complain, that the fault lies with the hasty ejaculation of the husband.[66]

The new view of women – which held that as far as conception was concerned it was of no importance how indifferent or indeed hostile they might be to the sexual act – did result in one unexpected reform. By the nineteenth century, courts dealing with rape cases no longer assumed that the pregnancy of the victim implied her acquiescence. 'It was formerly supposed', wrote E. H. East in 1803, 'that if a woman conceived it was no rape, because that showed her consent; but it is now admitted on all hands that such an opinion has no foundation either in reason or law'.[67]

Thus the medical literature depicts a change from the sexually active woman of the seventeenth century to the passionless creature of the nineteenth. The reasons for this are still under debate. Some writers have suggested that the rise of evangelical religion was responsible for the new stress on women's chastity, decorum and purity.[68] Others have argued that doctors rather than priests played a key role in counselling moderation – that purity and suspicion of sexuality were exploited by physicians in order to enhance their positions as counsellors and confessors.[69] Still others have suggested that the emergence of a new economic view of the world that lauded thrift, prudence and self-control necessarily influenced in a negative fashion sensual enjoyments.[70] Finally, some writers have argued that 'passionlessness' was in part a strategy seized upon by women to protect themselves from male sexual demands, specifically to limit pregnancies, but more generally as a means of allowing women at least a negative control over sexuality.[71] The purpose of this chapter has been to examine the role played in this evolution by medical scientists who were influenced by, but also obviously influenced, the other participants in the debate over sexuality. The main argument of this work is that the rights of women to sexual pleasure were not enhanced, but eroded as an unexpected consequence of the elaboration of more sophisticated models of reproduction.[72]

Why did doctors participate in the rejection of the old image of the lusty female and in the new portrayal of the solemnity and sacredness of procreation which required female sub-missiveness? Margaret Jacob, surprised to find that so many eighteenth-century scientists were religious and turned their ideas to support a natural theology, concluded that to under-stand the Newtonians one had to appreciate the extent to which they tailored their philosophy of nature to serve the social and political purposes of liberal, Protestant interests.[73] In a remark-ably similar fashion medical scientists appear to have turned the later eighteenth-century discussion of procreation to the purposes of bolstering a new, middle-class image of the respectable, asexual female.[74] The notion of aggressive, female sexuality did not disappear but would henceforth be associated by medical men only with working-class women. Doctors in this way contributed to the effort made on a variety of fronts by the middle classes to elaborate new social and sexual roles to differentiate their enlightened lives from the unthinking, hedonistic existences of both the upper and lower orders.

These conclusions bring into question the assertions of Stone, Shorter and Trumbach that the eighteenth century saw the dawning of a new era of sensual enjoyment. But while taking issue with the idea that the sexual pleasure of women was unknown in early modern Britain this study does not suggest that in contrast to the constrained Victorian world there once existed a Merrie Englande of 'uncontrolled' sexuality: what it does indicate is that in every century women's roles are prescribed and given elaborate medical and biological justifications. In the early nineteenth century it appeared subversive to argue that spouses had the same sexual needs, but from the sixteenth to the eighteenth centuries the commonplace assumption was made that the bed was one place at least in which men and women were more or less equal.[75] The view was fairly egalitarian but not entirely so given the fact that male physical and psychological needs were taken as the norm against which women's acts and feelings were measured. According to much of the popular literature all women were lascivious and amorous, and it must be recalled that in examining such texts we are gaining insights into what were often mere male fantasies about female sexuality. Nevertheless, a review of this literature suggests that it is a gross oversimplification to argue that love, affection and sexual enjoyment were unknown in the 'world we have lost'. This chapter has explained why the pleasure of the woman was believed in past times to have played an important part in ensuring conceptions; how such conceptions could be further promoted and protected is the subject of the following chapter.

2

'To remedy barrenness and to promote the faculty of generation': promoting fertility, 1500–1800

Motherhood [is] in each culture a relationship specific to that culture, different from all other motherhoods, and correlated to the whole social structure of the community.
Bronislaw Malinowski, *Sex, Culture, and Myth* (1930).

In linking pleasure and procreation early modern English men and women were indicating that they saw themselves playing an active role in reproduction. Though the forces of fertility were wrapped in mystery, spouses nevertheless saw themselves as being more than mere pawns blindly following iron laws of reproduction in some Malthusian demographic tragedy. Yet, if earlier generations did assume they enjoyed some power over reproduction how did they square their high fertility to this purported control of procreation? The question is anachronistic and unfair. In the twentieth century control of reproduction is equated with the driving down of the rate of fertility but 'birth control' can of course be manifested by a forcing up of the rates of fertility. It was the latter form of power over reproduction that figured most centrally in the sixteenth- and seventeenth-century writings on sexuality. In later chapters we shall return to the question of how one might seek to limit fertility; this chapter examines the complementary issue of how conceptions could be assured and miscarriages avoided.

To make intelligible a discussion of the ways in which past generations sought to promote their fertility it has to be noted that children were highly prized: by the religious as a sign of God's blessing; by the wealthy as an assurance of the continuation of the family line; by the poor as a possible source of security; by some women – who were proud of their sexuality and closely related it to their capacity to bear children – as a demonstration of the maternal power which established their status. The fact that most wives in early modern England bore a child within the first two years of marriage has been taken by some demographers as evidence of earlier generations' 'natural fertility'. But such a designation gives a completely false picture of the extent to which childbearing preoccupied women in the past. They regarded their fertility, not as 'natural', but as part of their social and cultural creation. Upon investigation one finds that the birth process was not left to fate, but marked at each stage by social rituals. From conception through gestation to birth early modern English spouses had at their disposal a vast range of traditional sexual lore that was of importance as much because of the reassurance it offered as for whatever medical benefit it might confer. They had elaborated a 'framework of explanation' in which the process of procreation lost much of its frightening mystery and became amenable to individual desires.

How each stage of the process from conception to birth could be most successfully navigated was explained in receipt books, popular sex manuals, traditional medical texts and common folklore. In this chapter the advice available to early modern men and women on the ways in which potential obstacles to childbearing could be overcome will be reviewed. How did humoral theories, in linking the psychological and the physiological, explain differences in fecundity? Which herbs could be used to provoke the lust and elicit the seed of the man? How were aphrodisiacs employed? To which potions should a barren woman turn? What were the magical causes of sterility? What were the physical? Which positions were most propitious for a fertile union? At what times were couples most fertile? How could one know if conception had occurred? If a boy or girl had been conceived? How could miscarriages be avoided? Were the longings of pregnant women dangerous? And, finally, how might the pains of labour be eased? To understand the ways in which the patterning of fertility was sought, each of these issues will be investigated in what follows.

Humoral theories

Children were highly prized in pre-industrial England. But what if a union were infertile? Medical writers discussed a variety of causes of sterility, including a lack of affection between spouses. Doctors paid such attention to emotion because scientific writers had linked the physiological and the psychological in their explanations of sexual malfunctioning. Underlying this approach to health was a humoral model of physiology based on four primary physical qualities: heat, cold, moisture and dryness. Excess heat and dryness, it was believed, led to anger, cold and dryness to sorrow, heat and moisture to sensuality, and so on. Love was associated with blood and the sanguine complexion. Seed was but distilled blood,

> made White by the Natural Heat, and an Excrement of the Third Digestion after the third and last concoction: . . . in everie part of the bodie that is nourished, there is left some part of the profitable bloud, not needefull to the partes, ordeyned by nature for procreation which . . . is woender-fullie conveighed and carried to the genitories, where by their proper nature that which before was plaine bloud, is now transformed and changed into seed.[1]

Because blood was being constantly distilled into seed, according to this theory, it followed that moderate sexual indulgence was necessary and healthy. But because seed was the most precious distillation of the blood, excessive indulgence was necessarily debilitating.[2] The body at birth was provided with a limited amount of heat and moisture which diminished over time, cooling and drying being equated in the traditional mind with the forces of death and decay. Therefore the hot and fiery young were, according to Robert Burton, 'most apt to love' but such passions had to be avoided by the aged.[3]

The humoral theory not only explained physiological function but also gave instructions on how sexual powers could be abetted. Sterility was, according to such theories, attributed to some imbalance in the humours that rendered either the man or woman too hot or too dry, too cold or too moist. Such imbalances could be remedied by bleedings, purges and special diets.[4] If, for example, barrenness was caused by lack of female heat, resulting in a 'slippery' womb, Lemnie and Newton advised a diet of rich meats to raise the temperature and guarantee conception.[5] Barrough likewise praised 'Meates that doe heate and engender good humours'. For women whose natures according to Galenic theory had to be cooler and wetter, moist meats like lamb and kid and leafy vegetables were recommended. Thus, in the words of Thomas Browne,

> in this way do all vegetables make fruitful according unto the complexion of the matrix; if that excel in heat, plants exceeding in cold do rectify it; if it be cold, simples that are hot reduce it; if dry, moist; if moist, dry correct it; in which division all plants are comprehended.[6]

For drier, hotter-natured men 'windy meates' like nuts, beans and scallions were prescribed.

How did one know which meats and vegetables to consume? Much of the dietary advice was based on common sense. If a person were 'cold' warming foods were necessary. Remedies, to the extent that they imitated nature, were assumed and appeared to work. Beyond such empirical responses, however, many herbalists and doctors subscribed to the theory of 'signatures' – the belief that plants carried a code indicating their nature and use. According to Coles every herb upon investigation indicated its appointed role, provided in each leaf a 'lecture in divinity', and thus proved the existence of God.[7] For example, walnuts (because of their shape) were useful for remedies of the head; white lilies indicated their ability to cure problems of the breast. Savin similarly had the signature of the veins of the matrix or womb; the kernels of the fistick nut (pistachio) the signature of the testicles; the bulbous root of satyrion suggested a power to provoke lust, the lank root to abate it; cotton seeds, by their numbers, to increase the seeds of generation. As their names implied, the birthwort and Ladies' Bedstraw were thought to ease delivery, while Ladies' Mantle helped in nursing as did Rampions which if the root were broken sent forth white juice 'which was an apparent signature' for engendering milk.[8] A general familiarity with such doctrines would mean that Shakespeare's audience understood, when, in Act II of *Romeo and Juliet*, Friar Laurence exclaims:

O, mickle is the powerful grace that lies
In plants, herbs, stones, and their true qualities.
For naught so vile that on the earth doth live
But to the earth some special good doth give. . .[9]

Herbal potions to counter male sterility

Armed with a knowledge of the humours, an appreciation of
the medicinal powers of plants as shown by their signatures,
and some understanding of astrological influences, it was
thought possible to make a person amorous and fecund
whether or not he or she was naturally sanguine. To provoke
the lusts of men and increase seed, herbalists prescribed a
variety of highly nutritive and frequently flatulent food. Ray's
collection of seventeenth-century proverbs included one that
advised:

He that would an old wife wed
Must eat an apple before he goes to bed.
(Which by its flatulency is apt to excite lust.)[10]

The list also included artichokes, almonds, cotton seeds, chest-
nuts, chocolate, wild carrots, clary, coriander, dragon's blood
(resin), dates, eringo (candied sea holly, a traditionally popular
aphrodisiac), fistick nuts, ginger, garlic, leeks, mustard,
nettles, peas, rocket, rue, sassafras, satyrion, scallions and
skirrets.[11] The aphrodisiac reputation of scallions stretched
back to the classical age. One of the epigrams of Martial warned
that

Scallions, lustful rockets nought prevail,
And heightening meats in operation fail;
Thy wealth begins the pure cheeks to defile,
So venery provoked lives but a while;
Who can admire enough, the wonder's such
That thy not standing stands thee in so much?[12]

Geoffrey Chaucer spoke in *The Merchant's Tale* of similar
recourse to sexual stimulants:

He drynketh ypocras, claree, and vernage
Of spices hoote, t'encressen his corage.[13]

Satyrion, a member of the orchid family, by its very name

35

suggested its employment. In his rendition of Chaucer, Alexander Pope presents the hero:

> The Foe once gone, our Knight prepar'd t'undress,
> So keen he was, and eager to possess:
> But first thought fit th'Assistance to receive,
> Which grave Physicians scruple not to give;
> *Satyrion* near, with hot *Eringo's* stood,
> *Cantharides*, to fire the lazy Blood,
> Whose Use old Bards describe in luscious Rhymes,
> And Criticks learn'd explain to Modern Times.[14]

In *The Soldier's Fortune* (1681) Thomas Otway has Sir Jolly serve both 'Ringoes' and Satyrion. Sir Jolly explains: 'odd 'tis the root Satyrion, a very pretious plant, I gather 'em every *May* my self, odd they'l make an old fellow of sixty-five cut a Caper like a Dancing Master'.[15] Falstaff was of similar appetites and at the end of *The Merry Wives of Windsor* calls out, 'Let it . . . hail kissing-comfits, and snow eringoes.'[16] John Dryden in his translation of Juvenal (1735) portrays libertines:

> Who lewdly dancing at a midnight ball
> For hot eryngoes and fat oysters call.[17]

If the name of satyrion suggested its employment so obviously did the 'Wild Rocket' which Langham and others claimed 'moveth Venus'. To 'cause standing of the yard' Sowerby recommended saffron; garlic was said to stir lust but unfortunately or fortunately, depending on the case, also dried up seed; according to William Turner, the father of English botany, clary 'stirreth men to the getting of children'; and coriander (which means 'much seed') 'provoketh a man to much venery'; skirret, it was said, 'stirreth a man to lechery'; and rue was discovered to have the unusual quality of provoking lust in a woman and abating it in a man.[18] Underlying the prescriptions of such diets was the belief that sexual failure on the man's part was usually attributable to cold, thin seed that required heat.

Aphrodisiacs

In the twentieth century the mention of the use of aphrodisiacs conjures up the image of scenes of seduction. In the early modern period their employment by the unmarried was cer-

tainly a concern. Othello was accused of employing 'philtres' to
capture the love of Desdemona:

> That thou has practis'd on her with foul charms,
> Abus'd her delicate youth, with drugs or minerals,
> That weakens motion . . .[19]

John Aubrey reported:

> Young wenches have a wanton sport which they call *moulding
> of Cocklebread: vis.* they get upon a Table-board, and then
> gather-up their knees and their Coates with their hands as
> high as they can then they wabble to and fro with their
> Buttocks as if they were kneading of Dowgh with their Arses,
> and say these words, *viz.*
>
>> 'My Dame is sick and gone to bed
>> And I'le go mowld my Cockle-bread.'
>
> I did imagine nothing to have been in this but meer
> Wantonnesse of Youth. . . . But I find in . . . Buchardus in his
> Methodus Confitendi on the VII Commandment, one of the
> articles of interrogating a young Woman is, if she did ever
> *subjgere panem clunibus*, and then bake it, and give it to the
> one she loved to eate. . . . So here I finde it to be a relique of
> Naturall Magick: an unlawful Philtrum.[20]

One of the characters in Beaumont and Fletcher's *Philastre*
(1610) says of a woman, 'before shee was common talke, now
none dare say Cantharides can stirre her'. And cantharides
(powdered blister beetles or Spanish Flies) were also the
weapon of a woman in John Gay's *The Shepherd's Week* (1714)
who confessed:

> Strait to the 'pothecary shop I went,
> And in *love powder* all my money spent;
> Behap what will, next Sunday after prayers,
> When to the alehouse Lubberkin repairs,
> These golden flies into his mug I'll throw,
> And soon the swain with fervent love shall glow.[21]

Interesting as such accounts of seduction are they can obscure
the fact that most of the references in the popular and medical
literature relate to the use of herbal potions by married couples
to increase fertility. The distinction between the two uses of

such potions is made especially clear when one turns to their employment by women.

Herbal potions to counter female barrenness

The problem of provoking lust was presented as mainly a male concern and one was clearly dealing with the issue of impotency. If the sexual act was successfully carried out but conception still did not follow then the assumption was usually made that the female was barren. Whether or not the woman was fertile could be tested; for example, by watering corn with her urine. If it grew she was not barren. If it did not, a variety of remedies were at hand to increase her fecundity.[22] Sea holly was recommended by Elizabeth Okeover; nutmeg would 'help conception and strengthen nature' asserted Miss Springatt; sitting over hot fumes of catmint was suggested by several authors.[23] Anything that warmed and invigorated such as brandy and hot baths found favour. Nicholas Culpeper, self-proclaimed student in physick and astrology, provided in his *Directory for Midwives* (1656) typically elaborate instructions on how to aid conception. In addition to good diet and exercise he recommended wearing amulets such as a lodestone or the heart of a quail; drinking potions of eringo, peony and satyrion; eating 'fruitful' creatures such as crabs, lobsters and prawns; and consuming concoctions of the dried and powdered wombs of hares, the brains of sparrows and the pizzles of wolves.[24]

The semi-magical basis of such advice is obvious. Katherine Boyle suggested that in order to remedy barrenness and promote the faculty of generation one should use the salt of mugwort, wear an amulet of carolina root and walk in the shadow of 'a strong lusty fruitful woman . . . so treading will attract the strength and fruitfulness of the other'.[25]

Mandrake was long reputed to have the most powerful magical reproductive powers because of its association with the Old Testament story of Rachel. In seventeenth-century Boston, John Winthrop wrote of one midwife who,

> used to give young women oil of Mandrakes and other Stuff to cause conception and she grew into great suspicion to be a witch, for it was creditably reported that, when she gave any medicines (for she practised physick), she would ask the party if she believed she could help her, etc.[26]

Other magical plants which were used in one way or another to stir up the passions included vervaine, smallage, mistletoe, angelica and elder leaves.[27]

Magical causes of barrenness

What were the particular magical causes of and cures for barrenness? It is difficult to separate magic and medicine in the period under discussion.[28] Herbs were supposed to be collected at certain times – for example during the full moon – and often while repeating specific prayers or charms so that their powers were always more than a mere consequence of their organic composition. Such potency was required because when all other explanations failed it was always possible to attribute barrenness to enchantments and spells.[29] Though demonologists agreed that the devil had no power over the organs of man there was one exception. 'The Devil by God's permission', wrote the authors of the *Malleus Maleficarum* (1488), 'has great power over the genital organs, for the serpent which trails over the earth signifies the serpent of lust'.[30] Of course, early modern English men and women were also aware that fears of magical impotency pre-dated Christianity. In John Dryden's translation of Ovid (1729) a man asks:

Is Verse, or Herbs the source of present Harms?
Am I a Captive of Thessalian Charms?
Has some Enchantress this Confusion brought;
And in soft Wax my tortur'd Image wrought?[31]

This is not the place to provide an extended discussion of witchcraft, but it has to be noted that fears of blighted fertility were the subject of the acts passed against witchcraft by the English Parliament in 1542, 1563 and 1604: the last statute was only revoked in 1736. It was believed that charms could be used either to provoke or destroy love. Thus in 1542 Parliament made it a felony punishable by a year in jail and exhibition in the pillory 'to provoke any persone to unlawfull love'.[32] In Thomas Dekker's *The Shoemaker's Holiday* (1599) June says to a man reputed to use love charms

I could be coy, as many women be,
Feed you with sunshine smiles and wanton looks,
But I detest witchcraft.[33]

Thomas Newton in *Tryall of a Man's Owne Selfe* (1602) asked his readers threateningly, 'Whether by any secret sleight, or cunning, as drinkes, drugges, medicines, *charmed potions, amatorious philters*, figures, characters, or any such like paltering instruments, devises, or practises, thou has gone about to procure others to doate for love of thee'.[34] Impotency was likewise attributed to the forces of witchcraft and on occasion such diabolically caused barrenness was used as grounds in petitions for divorce. Reginald Scot's *The Discoverie of Witchcraft* (1584) popularized in England the fears of sterile charms noted by the authors of *Malleus Maleficarum*:

> They also affirme, that the virtue of generation is impeached by witches both inwardlie and outwardlie: for intrinsicallie they repress the courage, and they stop the passage of the mans seed, so as it may not descend to the vessels of generation: also they hurt extrinsicallie, with images, hearbs, etc.[35]

Scot recommended for those 'bewitched in the privie members' the breathing in of the smoke of the tooth of a dead man, anointing oneself with the gall of a crow, spitting in one's own bosom and pissing through a wedding ring. Simon Forman, the astrological physician, as well as making up protective potions and sigils, provided similar advice for such problems.[36]

In Forman's works we also find references to the use of the magical ligature or knotted cord to render couples infertile. Le Roy Ladurie has chronicled the belief in castration by magic in France in the sixteenth century.[37] A full contemporary discussion of such magic was provided by the eminent political theorist and demonologist Jean Bodin. He found that a leather cord could be tied in such a way so as to restrict the fertility of one or both spouses for any length of time, and to render them either impotent or simply barren. The spell was cast usually at the marriage itself by a participant who secretly knotted the cord with the words 'Whom God hath joined together let the Devil separate.'[38] Some doctors refused to treat such cases of barrenness as beyond their competence. For example, the famous French surgeon, Ambroise Paré, set aside all barrenness caused by 'inchantment, magick, witching, and enchanted knots, bands and ligatures, for those causes belong not to physick, neither may they bee taken away by the remedies of our art'.[39] In England, Francis Bacon was one of the first to note the practice but his reports were drawn from the continent: 'In Zant it is very ordinary to make men impotent to accompany with their wives. The like is practised in Gascony; where it is called *nouer l'equillette*. It is practised always upon the wedding-day'.[40] Robert Burton included the ligature in his list of 'diabolical means' to affect the psyche: 'by Spells, cabalistic words, Charmes, Characters, Images, Amulets, Ligatures, Philtures, Incantations, etc'.[41] The employment of such a knot was a central theme in Thomas Heywood and Richard Brome's *The Late Lancashire Witches* (1634). When the newly married Lawrence proves impotent, Squire Doughty suspects the bride: 'Witchery, witchery, more witcherie still flate and plaine witchery. Now do I thinke upon the codpiece point the young jade gave him at the wedding; shee is a witch, and that was a charme, if there be any in the world'.[42] Nicholas Culpeper thought cures were possible. After dealing with the issue of 'natural barrenness' which could be cured by various herbal remedies he turned to the problem of 'Barrenness against nature':

> It is not one Physicians Opinion alone, That many Women are made Barren by Diabolical means. I do not call them Diabolical, because they cannot be acted without invocation of evil Spirits, but because they are done by abuse of Nature; for as the right use of Natural things is from God, so the abuse of them is from the Devil. And so many unworthy creatures are wont to serve men and women at the very time of their Marriage, that the Man can never (before it is remedied) have to do carnally with his Wife. However to prevent such mischief, Authors have left waies.[43]

The 'waies' noted by Culpeper included wearing a St John's Wort, the heart of a turtle dove, a lodestone, or hanging over the bed a whole squill. If a man could still not give his wife 'due benevolence' he could be cured by 'making water through his Wifes Wedding-Ring'.

Jane Sharp in *The Compleat Midwife's Companion*, originally published in 1671 and reprinted in 1725, repeated the advice of pissing through the wedding ring.[44] *The Compleat Midwife* (1663) recognized that barrenness could be caused by 'inchantments: and then the man cannot lye with his wife; or, though he should, yet cannot emit the seed', and claimed that drinking the drops of water falling from the mouth of a stallion or stone-horse could act as a cure.[45] John Webster in *The Displaying of*

41

Supposed Witchcraft (1677), a largely sceptical analysis of purported magical feats, found it strange that people continued in
the late seventeenth century to talk of 'Ligation or binding of
husbands that they might not be viripotent, or be able to have
to do with their Wives'.[46] But Webster also made the interesting
comment that some women used such magic for their own
purposes: 'it is often performed by the Mothers to prevent that
incantation by others, and that they may loose it when they
please'. Francis Bacon had made the same observation: 'And in
Zant the mothers themselves do it [employ magical knots] by
way of prevention; because thereby they hinder other charms,
and can undo their own'.[47] Today in East Africa, Yao women go
to a special knot-tier who produces a ligature out of tree bark. It
ensures barrenness until the woman wishes to conceive. Then,
'she unties the knots, submerges the cord in water, drinks the
water, and throws the cord away'.[48] Magic can thus be used
against magic. The symbolisms of both are fairly obvious.
Knotting was equated to castration and urinating through the
wedding ring to intercourse. Did the knots 'work'? Bacon made
the perceptive comment that they could have some psychological effect, 'which must be referred to the imagination of him
that tieth the point. I conceive it to have less affinity with
witchcraft, because not peculiar persons only, (such as witches
are,) but any body may do it'.[49] That they were taken seriously
is indicated by the fact that in 1705 two persons in Scotland
were condemned to death for stealing knots to harm the
wedded happiness of Spalding of Ashintilly, and in France, as
late as 1718, the Parlement of Bordeaux had a knot-maker burnt
alive.[50]

Other semi-magical responses to barrenness included the
wearing of amulets or talismanic devices. Coral – presumably
because of its resemblance to myriads of tiny eggs – was long
popularly reputed to elicit fertility.[51] It was possibly ground
coral that made up the powder that Mary Woods in 1613 gave
the Countess of Essex to wear round her neck in order to
conceive.[52] Aetites or eaglestone (a sort of 'pregnant' pebble of
hollow ironstone with a loose nucleus, purportedly found in
eagles' nests, to which were ascribed medical and magical
properties) was also highly esteemed. Lemnie in 1658 reported:

It makes women that are slippery able to conceive, being
bound to the wrist of the left arm, by which from the heart

toward the ring finger, next to the little finger, an artery runs; and if all the time the woman is great with child this jewel be worn on those parts, it strengthens the child, and there is no fear of abortion or miscarrying.[53]

Similarly Coles in 1656 claimed, 'The seeds of Dock tyed to the left arme of a Woman, doe helpe Barrennesse'.[54] The talismanic devices could consist of characters, charms and prayers written on scraps of paper and worn on the person. Almost all the references we have to them by the seventeenth century are censorious.[55] Dr Jacques Ferrand in *Love Melancholy* (1640) condemned charms, 'such as no Christian physician ought to use; notwithstanding that the common people doe to this day too superstitiously believe and put in practice many of these paganish devices'.[56] In *Mag-Astromancers Posed and Puzzl'd* (1651), John Gaule asked, 'whether pericepts, amulets, prae-fiscinals, phylacteries, niceteries, ligatures, suspensions, charms, and spells, had ever been used, applyed or carryed about, but for magick and strologie'.[57] Henry Bourne in 1725 cited Bingham:

> To this kind belong all ligatures, and remedies, which the schools of physitians reject and condemn; whether in inchantments or in certain marks, which they call characters, or in some other things which are to be hanged and bound about the body.[58]

By the late seventeenth and early eighteenth century it was becoming obvious that the magical awe of reproduction was beginning to decline. The 1694 edition of *Aristotle's Masterpiece* tartly observed, 'Many there are that conceive Barrenness is frequently caused by Inchantation, but these Opinions are altogether frivolous and vain'.[59] But the very fact that so many writers felt compelled to continue to attack such beliefs suggests that they had a greater tenacity than is usually allowed.

Physical causes of barrenness

Writers on sexuality also noted that physical causes of barren-ness could exist. It was believed by some that if the veins behind the ears were cut, the blood from the brain needed to produce seed could not flow.[60] More common was the assump-tion that spouses had to be of a generally complementary stature: they should not be too short or too tall, too thin or too fat. The womb should not be too straight or bent nor the man's 'yard' too short. Addressing the latter problem, Barrough stated that some were so small 'so that they can not cast their seede into the innermost place of the matrice, which also sometimes chaunceth through fatnesse: for fat men have such great bellies, that they cannot cast their seed into the deepest partes of the bodies'.[61] Fatness could be brought about by idleness and luxury which some held to provoke lust. Timothy Bright in *A Treatise on Melancholie* (1586) asserted that the indolent were more given to venery than the labouring poor because labour lowered the heat of the body and consumed the spirit.[62] Robert Burton in his better-known *Anatomy of Melancholy* (1621) agreed that the 'aptest to love are those that are young and lusty, live at ease, stall-fed, free from cares, like cattle in rank pasture'.[63] But others held that the life-style of the upper orders was in fact a detriment to reproduction. Navarro declared in 1594 that procreation was governed by exercise,

> for this fretteth and consumeth the excessive moisture of the seed, and heateth and drieth the same. By this means a man becommeth most fruitful and able for generation: and contrariwise to give our selves to our ease, and not to exercise the bodie, is one of the things which breedeth most coldnes and moisture in the seed. Therefore rich and dainty persons, are lesse charged with children, than the poor who take pains.[64]

As proof of his assertion Navarro pointed to the fact that the Israelites, though in bondage, outbred the Egyptians. The anonymous author of *The Family Companion for Health* (1729) held the upper classes' penchant for hunting as specifically responsible for their barrenness because it 'consumes the Spirits and bruises the virile Parts. . . . Hunting is a prejudicial Exercise for such as long for Children; the Poor therefore, are more burden'd with children than the Rich'.[65] Thomas Percival, at the end of the eighteenth century, acknowledged that 'Luxury, when carried to such a degree as to enervate the constitution, is unfavourable to population'.[66]

Positions and timing of intercourse

In the traditional texts advice on the mechanics of sex was limited. As far as positions were concerned it was generally assumed that only one was natural. According to Venette, 'Nature has taught both Sexes such Postures as are allowable; and that contribute to Generation; and Experience has shown those that are forbidden and Contrary to Health'.[67] The man was supposed to be uppermost but for legitimate reasons, for example, a wife's pregnancy, it was considered permissible for him to enter from the side or the back. The idea of the woman on top particularly enraged authors like Venette who warned that any possible children of such unions were likely to be, 'Dwarfs, Cripples, Hunch-back'd, Squint ey'd, and stupid Blockheads, and by their Imperfections would fully evidence the irregular Life of their Parents, without putting us to the trouble to search the Cause of such Defects any further'.[68] The readers of *Aristotle's Masterpiece* were further cautioned that they should separate slowly and carefully after the act and that the woman should avoid 'both coughing and sneezing, both which are great hindrances to conception after the Act of Copulation'.[69]

With regard to the timing of intercourse, a range of advice was given. Plato recommended sex once a week; Willich in 1794 suggested three to four times a week.[70] All authors warned that too-frequent intercourse led to debility. Robert Burton gave the problem his usual serious consideration:

> The extremes being both bad, the medium is to be kept, which cannot easily be determined. Some are better able to sustaine, such as hote and moist, phlegmatick as *Hippocrates* insinuateth, some strong and lusty, well fed like *Hercules*, *Proclus* the Emperor, *Messalina* the Empresse, and by Philters, and such kinde of lascivious meates, use all meanes to inable themselves and brag of it: others impotent, of a cold and dry constitution cannot sustaine those gymnasticks without great hurt done unto their owne bodies, of which number are melancholy men for the most part.[71]

Bunworth in 1656 argued that whores did not reproduce because their wombs were 'slippery' as a result of overuse.[72] Fontanus asserted that respectable wives could suffer the same fate.[73] Early marriages were, it was thought, often without issue because the seed of the spouses was still too weak and thin; the same was asserted of the elderly. There was general agreement that the days following a woman's period were the most fertile and when one was most likely to conceive male children whereas in the second week after menstruation one would conceive girls. It was also, naturally enough, assumed that the warm, moist months of spring, the 'vernal months', were most conducive to fruitful unions, while the hot, dry months of late summer were not.[74]

Determination of pregnancy and sex of offspring

Assuming all went well by the second month of gestation most women would, because of nausea, increased breast size and cessation of the menses, realize they were pregnant. But some authors claimed that at the very moment of conception a woman might know that she had conceived because of a sudden sense of sickness or an unexpected bout of shivering.[75] Sermon informed his readers that the man could also tell that conception had occurred by feeling a sucking sensation on the yard.[76] From the time of Hippocrates pregnant women were said to lose their sense of smell, failing to recognize, for example, garlic. Stronger indicators of pregnancy were offered by uroscopy. In Owen Wood's *An Alphabetical Book of Physical Secrets* (1639) it was claimed that if, after boiling, a woman's urine was 'red as gold with a watery circle above' it 'shows she is with child'; the same was true if she could see her face in it; if the urine was white the child was dead; if there were clear streaks in it, it was evidence that the 'childe hath life'.[77] Katherine Boyle, however, gave the opposite diagnosis: urine boiled with salt which turned white indicated a pregnancy; a red colour did not.[78]

A range of tests was also employed to try to determine the sex of the child. John Cotta cited Hippocrates to the effect that if the woman's right breast was firmer, or her right eye brighter, she would have a boy; if the left, a girl.[79] Cold food was reputed to favour the formation of girls; warm food, boys. Guillemeau repeated the belief that younger mothers more frequently had males and older mothers females. Equally popular was the conviction that boys sat higher in the womb than girls, a belief that has lasted on into the twentieth century.[80]

Protection from miscarriage

Once conception was assured the next task was to take all possible measures to avoid miscarrying. In the 1980s still something like a third of all conceptions are spontaneously terminated. The rate of miscarriages and consequent complications for the mother's health was appreciably more important in the early modern period. Lawrence Stone estimates that the chance of a wife dying in the first fifteen years of marriage was twice that of her spouse's.[81] This explains why so much advice was given on the subject. Protection was offered, authors suggested, by a great variety of strategies ranging from the mundane to the magical. Some of it sounds quite modern. Women were told to avoid strenuous exercise, moderate their diets, sleep as much as possible and abstain from tight corseting.[82] Whether or not the exercise of conjugal rights during pregnancy was dangerous was debated. Sermon said that in the first four months it certainly was dangerous and in any event women, 'when they are with child, hate to accompany with their husbands'.[83] Animals abstained during gestation but man, lamented Walter Harris, 'almost more salacious than a *Buck-Goat*, not knowing how to restrain and bridle his Lust, importuneth his Mate from her first Conceiving until the hour of Birth'.[84] Others disagreed and Pechey went so far as to assert that intercourse in the latter months 'is thought to facilitate delivery'.[85]

A variety of strengthening herbs and potions was passed on from woman to woman. In the receipt books of the landed classes, for example, are references to 'A powder for a woman that is likely to miscarry – dragons blood as much as will lie on a grote', and 'A receipt to prevent miscarrying sent to my sister Cartwright by her niece the Duchess of Buckingham'.[86] Such cordials – frequently consisting of cinnamon, nutmeg, sugar and eggs – were aimed at warming and strengthening the mother-to-be. Tansy also had a reputation as a protective.[87] A seventeenth-century author claimed that if applied to the belly it prevented miscarriage; in the eighteenth century another writer asserted 'Let those women that desire children love this herb, it is their best companion, their husband excepted'.[88]

Religious and magical devices also found a place in preventing miscarriage just as they did in ensuring conception. Safety was sought by some in amulets. Johanna St John suggested that one take 'a dryed toad and hang it about the waist'.[89] An eaglestone worn about the neck was supposed to protect against miscarriage and, tied to the thigh, to ease the birth. Magnets, lodestones and jasper were all reputed to have similarly protective properties.[90] Walter Harris writing in 1683 attacked the continued use of amulets and charms but conceded that an 'Eagle's Stone worn about the breast of a Breeding Woman, may thus be a means to Preserve her from Miscarrying' simply because she thought it would.[91]

Various girdles were also considered to be efficacious. A 1703 work mentioned a 'cerecloth to prevent abortion' containing wax and quinces and girdles of seahorse skin and wolfskin.[92] In the seventeenth century Ann Brumwich recommended wearing a piece of beaten lead on the navel and another on the small of the back while John Hall suggested a leather girdle applied to the loins and belly.[93] These girdles were supposed to support and protect the foetus, but they also had a religious significance in that they were modelled on the girdle of the virgin. Such girdles were passed on from mother to daughter along with the injunction to pray to St Margaret and St Edine for assistance in birth.[94] The upper orders were increasingly sceptical if not hostile to such traditions based on the idea that women were especially susceptible to the forces of evil during childbearing. John Bale in his *Comedye Concernynge Thre Lawes, Moses and Christ* (1538) noted that some women sought to employ charms and relics to assure their fertility:

> In Parys we have the mantell of St. Lewes,
> Which women seke moch, for help of their barrenness:
> For be it ones layed upon a wommanys bellye,
> She go thens with chylde, the miracles are seene there
> daylye.[95]

But such magical intervention, warned Bale, could be employed by the midwife in idolatrous fashion. He has one declare,

> Yea but now ych am a she
> And a good MYDWYFE perde
> Younge chyldren can I *charme*,
> With whysperynges and whysshynges,
> With crossynges and with Kyssinges,
> With blasynges and with blessynges,
> That spretes do them no harme.[96]

To counter the danger of the midwife becoming a witch or employing magic the 1554 Injunction of the Visitation of Edmonde, Bishop of London, declared, 'A mydwyfe (of the diocese and jurisdiction of London) shal not use or exercise any witchecrafte, charmes, sorcerye, invoications or praiers, other than suche as be allowable and may stand with the lawes and ordinances of the Catholike Churche'.[97] To track down those who might use magic to blight the fertility of their neighbours an inquiry was ordered in 1559 to determine 'whether you know any that doe use charmes, sorcery, enchauntementes, invoications, circles, witchcraftes, southsayinge, or any lyke craftes or imaginacions invented by the devyl, and specially in the tyme of women's travaylle'.[98] But though many midwives were ultimately persecuted as witches, the employment of charms during pregnancy continued well into the eighteenth century. Describing the popularity of an eaglestone in the seventeenth century, Dr Bargrave, Dean of Christchurch, Canterbury, stated:

> It is so useful that my wife can seldom keep it at home, and therefore she hath sewed the strings to the knitt purse in which the stone is, for the convenience of the tying it to the patient on occasion, and hath a box to put the purse and stone in. It were fitt that either the Dean's (Canterbury) or vice-dean's wife (if they be marryed men) should have this stone in their custody for the public good, as to neighbourhood; but still, that they have a great care into whose hand it be committed, and that the midwives have a care of it, so that it shall be the Cathedral's stone.[99]

This passage is of interest for two reasons. First, it reveals that the church tolerated and supported some forms of superstition. Second, it reveals, as do the receipt books of women of the gentry, that members of the upper orders frequently assumed the task of providing for lying-in women the potions and amulets they might need. Thus the assumption that such exotic items as eaglestones and expensive spices such as cinnamon and nutmeg were employed by only a tiny elite is not necessarily true.[100]

Force of the mother's imagination

During her pregnancy the woman was expected to have unusual desires and cravings. Walter Harris asserted that the diseases carried by the offspring were often the result of such manias: 'For *Teeming Women* are obnoxious to a thousand

49

Faults and Errors in their Diet'.[101] But such criticisms were moderated by the belief that if a woman's desires were frustrated the resulting anger could result in miscarriage. Accordingly, the mother's imagination was seen as a potent force 'which operates as a sort of seal stamping the image of the mother's fancy on the child she has conceived in the womb'.[102] Stories were told, for example, of the woman who deprived of a peach gave birth to a child with a 'peach' birthmark. Therefore, to prevent such problems husbands were told by doctors to dote on their spouses. Witkowski related that the celebrated botanist, Camerarius, was told by his pregnant wife that she felt an overwhelming desire to smash a dozen eggs in his face which he dutifully endured.[103] The liminal position of the woman thus provided her with some powers to compensate, however feebly, for the biological risks she ran. In the early eighteenth century a campaign was led by Blondel and others against the belief that the mother's imagination could in any way affect conception, sexual determination of the child and skin colouring.[104] Some of the mystery of gestation was accordingly lost and in the process some of the mythical powers of maternity.

Assistance during delivery

Once labour began the woman could expect to receive advice from friends and relatives on how to have an easy birth. In the medical texts and household books were lists of recipes for potions to aid labour or the 'throwes'. Wine, brandy and a variety of spices found their adherents.[105] A draft of breast milk was suggested by several authors.[106] These concoctions had as their main purpose the strengthening of the woman while the child forced its way into the world. Its passivity in the birth process was only established by Smellie in 1773.[107] Many herbs were employed specifically to precipitate delivery. Savin was the most powerful. *The Grete Herbal* of 1526 described savin as 'good to cause a chylde come out of its moders wombe' and a herbal of 1568 concurred that it 'dryve furth also the byrth'.[108] Pennyroyal 'provokes termes, easeth labour, takes afterbirth', reported other authorities.[109] Enjoying similar properties were wild thyme, wood bettony, birthwort, stinking arrach, Ladies' Bedstraw, horehound, angelica, bal, vervain, mugwort and cockle. In addition to potions, something very much like breathing exercises seems to be recommended by Barrough in 1652, in a section on avoidance of pain in childbirth: 'And if she was unskillfull of pains in travell admonish her to hold and stop her breath strongly, and let her thrust it out to the ilions [flanks] with all her might'.[110] It was commonly believed that by relaxing the pelvic region the birth pains could be eased. A sixteenth-century text followed the heading 'Against the payne in chylde birth' with a recipe for an ointment with which to 'annoint privities', Mrs Owen suggested hog's grease for the purpose, while Mrs Acton laconically dictated, 'To ease a woman big with child – straddle a pot of boiling sea water'.[111]

If labour still proved difficult recourse to magic might be made. The ringing of church bells was thought by some to aid in delivery.[112] More common was the belief that locks and knots in the vicinity of the woman might sympathetically impede the birth. For this reason, according to Pliny, the Romans thought it dangerous to sit by a woman in travail with crossed legs or clasped hands. G. L. Kittredge has noted,

> It is a widespread belief that when a woman is in labour, all knots must be untied and all locks unlocked. This piece of sympathetic magic is well-known to savage men. In New Guinea should labour be unduly prolonged, the child's father is sent for. He, after having opened any boxes there may be in the house . . . sits down near his wife and proceeds to untie the cord which confines her hair, and to remove the *gana* from his arm.[113]

So too we find that the Visitation of the Commissary of St Mary's, Salop in 1584 asked: 'Whether any mydwife within your parishe in tyme of weomens travill be knowne or suspected to use sorcerie, witchcrafte, charmes, unlockynge of chests and dores, . . . or to saye unlaweful praiers of superstitious invocations'.[114] Locks and knots were seen as impeding both easy births and easy deaths. As late as 1863 a Taunton jury of matrons at the bedside of a terminally ill child had all the locks and doors of the house opened to prevent him from 'dying hard'.[115]

If the birth were a success the woman might have recourse to featherfew to strengthen the womb, expel the afterbirth or secondine and remedy 'such infirmities as a careless midwife hath thereby caused'.[116] For after pains Mrs Cotton approved of balm water, pennyroyal, histeric water and mugwort. If the child was dead it could be expelled by potions of sage, ground pine, savin, pennyroyal, mugwort, tansy and birth tree. For the same problem Johanna St John asserted, 'the milk of another woman drunk helps presently'.[117] 'Let women drink ye juice of Rue', advised Langham, 'withe Wine to purge them after their deliverance and to expel the secondines, the dead childe, and unnaturalle birth'.[118]

Reproductive rituals or vulgar errors?

Social rituals thus marked each stage of the reproductive process. From conception through gestation to birth early modern English men and women exploited a vast range of traditional sexual lore that was of importance as much because of the reassurance it offered as for whatever medical benefit it might confer. They had elaborated a 'framework of explanation' in which the process of procreation lost much of its frightening mystery and became amenable to individual desires.

For a literary recapitulation of the tactics a young wife intent on childbearing might pursue, one can turn to *The Ten Pleasures of Matrimony* (1682), attributed to Aphra Behn. If, after several months of marriage, a conception had not occurred the impatient wife would, according to Behn, shamelessly discuss the most intimate details of her marital life with her female friends. After receiving their well-considered – though often contradictory – advice she would feed up her husband on the appropriate aphrodisiacs such as oysters, sweetbreads and chocolate, take physic herself and, to arouse her husband further, adopt 'pretty wanton postures'. If such activities went unrewarded the determined spouse could be understandably forgiven for calling her husband 'a John Cannot . . . a Fumbler, a dry-boots, and a good man Do-little'. The next step was to consult apothecaries, midwives, French doctors and Culpeper. Once again women friends would assist; 'then to work they go with smearing, annointing, chafing, infusing'. The fact that the woman finally proved with child did not end this feminine interference with the processes of procreation. Behn proceeds to detail the advice sought and given on the problems of the woman's 'longings', the pains of her labours, the plasters employed 'to raise the milk', and the stratagems to avoid the now inconvenient sexual demands of the husband.

This merry account of childbearing concludes with a 'gossip's feast' after the churching of the young mother. The women congratulate themselves – not the impersonal forces of nature – for bringing about the happy delivery of the mother and child.[119]

Eighteenth-century doctors, who were increasingly preoccupied by the dangers posed by irregular practitioners, not surprisingly attacked such continued involvement of women in health care. The elimination of the old crone who 'interfered' in the process of parturition would, they asserted, serve the interests of the State in protecting children, of mothers in assuring adequate aid and of the medical fraternity in removing professional rivals. William Cadogan in his influential *An Essay Upon Nursing* (1748) argued that 'the Preservation of Children should become the Care of Men of Sense because this business has been too long fatally left to the Management of Women'. He went on to attack 'the superstitious Practices and Ceremonies' which women inherited from their great-grandmothers, and warned men, 'I . . . earnestly recommend it to every Father to have his Child nursed under his own Eye, to make use of his own Reason and Sense'.[120] William Heberden asserted it was the doctor's duty to rescue children from the 'vulgar errors of old women and ignorant practitioners'.[121] Following the same line of argument James Nelson sneered at mothers' 'amazing Attachment to Nurses and what they call good Old Women'.[122] James Adair in *Medical Cautions* (1786) devoted a special chapter to denigrating the activities of 'Lady Doctors' whom he portrayed as all still reading and relying on such classics as '*Aristotle's Master-piece, Culpeper's Midwifery, Salmon's Practice of Physic,* and *Every Man his own Physician*'.[123] James Parkinson attacked as 'presumptuous nurses' those respectable countrywomen who doled out medicine to the local poor: 'At present it too frequently happens, that persons of influence and property are too much disposed, with the help of a family medicine chest, and a treatise on domestic medicine, to become the dispensers of physic to all their poor neighbours'.[124] If such ladies really wanted to help, declared Parkinson, they could best do so by contributing funds to the local lying-in hospital.

In part because of the attacks of doctors the marvellous armoury of potions, charms and amulets employed to assure conception and prevent miscarriage was subjected by the

enlightened to increased ridicule from the mid-seventeenth
century onwards and by the mid-eighteenth century occupied
a central place in accounts of the superstitions and popular
errors of the masses.[125] In John Arbuthnot and Alexander
Pope's *Martinus Scriblerus* (1741), the hero's father's vain
attempts to impregnate his wife is the occasion for a satiric
account of traditional beliefs:

> This [failure] was the utmost grief to the good man; especially
> considering what exact Precautions and Methods he used to
> procure that Blessing: For he never had cohabitation with his
> spouse, but that he ponder'd on the Rules of the Ancients, for
> the generation of Children of Wit. He ordered his diet
> according to the prescription of Galen, confining himself and
> his wife for almost the whole first year to Goat's Milk and
> Honey. It unfortunately befel her, when she was about four
> months gone with child, to long for somewhat which that
> author inveighs against, as prejudicial to the understanding
> of the Infant: This her husband thought fit to deny her,
> affirming, it was better to be childless than to become the
> Parent of a Fool. His wife miscarried; but as the Abortion
> proved only a female foetus, he comforted himself, that, had
> it arrived to perfection, it would not have answer'd his
> account; his heart being wholly fixed upon the learned Sex.[126]

Some historians of medicine have treated such customs with
the same disdain. For example, Audrey Eccles, the author of a
very useful history of obstetrics and gynaecology in the early
modern period, states that the best that can be said of popular
birthing beliefs is that they were usually harmless.[127] Such
authors ask simply whether the herbal remedies or charms
'worked', conclude that they did not, and leave out of consideration the emotional and cultural factors involved.
Historians may thus overlook the real care and reassurance that
was provided by recourse to such stratagems. In so doing they
also discount the importance of a woman's culture in which
mutual aid during pregnancy played such a central role.

There is of course a real danger of romanticizing the birth
experiences of earlier generations – experiences that were often
painful and dangerous. Some medical historians have been
eager to agree with the eighteenth-century medical men that
the interference of ignorant and untrained midwives led to
disastrous haemorrhaging and inverted uteri.[128] The point has

to be made, however, that the medical scientists of the 1700s, though they might pride themselves on their expertise in dealing with difficult deliveries, and contemptuously dismiss the myths and beliefs of old women, in normal deliveries they had little better to offer. The purpose of this chapter in examining the taboos, injunctions, charms and herbal potions employed to effect the process of gestation has not been to gloss over the very real fears women had when facing childbirth. Rather the intent is to show that because of the great import-ance of childbearing an accordingly complex framework of explanation was elaborated to deal with it.

This chapter argues that the traditional beliefs and customs deserve serious consideration. What they reveal is that early modern men and women did not have a rigid, mechanical view of reproduction. They perceived it as mutable – conditioned by diet, exercise, potions and charms.[129] The biological and cultural factors were seen by them as interacting in a way that their nineteenth-century descendants, dazzled by the apparent powers of biological determinism, often ignored. Twentieth-century demographers who employ the phrase 'natural fert-ility' – meaning the fertility of a population that does not use contraceptive techniques – may lose sight of this dialectical relationship. The married couples discussed in this chapter would be described by the demographer as having a 'natural fertility', but the anthropologist or cultural historian who takes note of the myriad rules and regulations, beliefs and fears that went into their procreative practices would respond that far from being 'natural' their fertility was a social and cultural creation.[130] It is understandable that the enlightened middle class of the eighteenth century would dismiss traditional sexual folklore as an indication of popular credulity and ignorance; historians who adopt the same stance fail to appreciate the complex view past people had of the world and their place in it.

Conception and birth continued to enjoy a magical aura in the early modern period. The Church sustained this image by blessing not only marriages and christenings but by offering its services during pregnancy to ward off miscarriage and at the time of 'churching' when the new mother was re-established in the public community.[131] But if procreation was an enchanted act it was possibly more so for the man than for the woman who bore the full burden of pregnancy and birth. The older medical writers in perceiving and deriding the barrenness of the

55

woman as a sort of sickness provided sanctions against those who might seek to avoid childbearing. Similarly, the rewards of increased status offered to the fruitful served to lure women into pregnancy. The number of rewards and punishments employed to maximize the reproductive powers of women further supports the view that their fertility was far from 'natural'.[132] Indeed it implies that the avoidance of child-bearing was also a real option, an issue to which we will turn in the following chapters.

3
'Excellent recipes to keep from bearing children': restricting fertility, 1500–1800

In Tikopia here when a married pair have an abundant family,
they stop, and manipulate things so that they are left on the
thighs.
Pa Tekaumata talking to Raymond Firth, *We, The Tikopia* (1936)

In a recent review of demographic literature Knodel and van de
Walle declared that all the available quantitative material
suggests that prior to the nineteenth century conscious
attempts to control fertility were of minimal importance:
'indirect evidence leads us to conclude that family limitation
was not a form of behavior known to the majority prior to the
fertility transition and thus not a real option for couples'. But,
like others in the field who are of the opinion that 'the adoption
of contraception within marriage occurred suddenly and
massively' in the latter half of the nineteenth century, Knodel
and van de Walle are primarily concerned with the numbers of
children born – not with the concerns and preoccupations of
their parents.[1] For the twentieth-century observer birth control
is usually taken to mean limitation of numbers. The fact that
high fertility norms were common in early modern England
might therefore be taken as proof that men and women in
earlier times had little interest in controlling births. Indeed
some scholars have argued that until recently the limitation of
fertility was 'unthinkable'.[2] Others believe that even if earlier
generations wanted to limit their fertility they could not have
done so because they lacked the necessary technology. To
demonstrate that this was not the case in early modern England

we shall in this chapter first review the discussion of family limitation prior to the nineteenth century and in the second and longer part of the chapter turn to the actual methods employed in the past to limit births. The argument is not that in past times the practices and purposes of controlling births were the same as those of the twentieth century. On the contrary, close examination reveals that it was not just how many children were born that concerned earlier communities but who had them, when, how far apart and up to what age.[3] The previous chapter provided evidence of the enormous amount of attention paid by couples to the ways in which conceptions could be assured and miscarriages avoided. This same knowledge of how to promote fertility could be applied to its restriction.

One can trace a long debate waged in the western world over the morality of the restriction of fertility. The debate is of importance for two reasons: it provides evidence that child-bearing was always regarded as problematical and, in shifting its terms of reference, reveals something of the differing moral and social preoccupations of different eras.

In the Middle Ages deliberate limitation of births was criticized on religious grounds. Churchmen were naturally the most vociferous critics of sterility, but as recent investigators have noted it was often the magic and superstition involved in contraceptive techniques, as much as non-procreative intercourse *per se*, that were the real targets of their diatribes. The very number of penitentials referring to contraception and abortion, moreover, seriously undermines the argument that earlier generations were ignorant of such basic forms of birth control as coitus interruptus.[4] The Reformation, by increasing access to the Bible, might even have served to expand the knowledge of Onan's sin. For those who missed the nuances of the tale Luther explained:

> Onan goes in to her [Tamar]; that is, he lies with her and copulates, and when it comes to the point of insemination, spills the semen, lest the woman conceive. Surely at such a time the order of nature established by God in procreation should be followed. Accordingly it was a most disgraceful crime to produce semen and excite the woman, and to frustrate her at that very moment.[5]

The sin, as far as Luther and the English Puritans were concerned, was not so much the method; rather it was the evidence thereby made of lack of faith and obedience. Children were declared by God to be a glory and blessing. To prevent their appearance by whatever means could be seen as a direct flouting of God's intention. Evidence that such disobedience was endemic is found in sixteenth- and seventeenth-century religious texts. Christopher Hooke in *The Child-birth or Woman's Lecture* (1590) declared that the importance of childbearing had to be stressed constantly:

> And this that it is so, is a most necessarie doctrine in these daies to be taught, in respect of . . . [those] who thinketh Children to be a charge: and therefore if they might have their choice, had rather to be without them than have them . . . by reason of their ignorant hearts, which never were instructed in Gods schoole, they take more comfort in the increase of their swine, than they do in the increase of sonnes and daughters.[6]

In the following century Thomas Hilder in *Conjugall Counsell* (1653) continued the argument that to avoid children was to violate God's command:

> Then by the way, it may be a word of just reproofe to many Men and Women that are afraid of Marriage lest they should have Children; as also of divers who are married, that use all meanes possible to prevent great increase of Children.

What 'means' Hilder had in mind he made clear when he added, 'I beseech you seriously to mind the sin, and punishment of a bird of your own feather, (viz) *Onan*, Gen. 38.9.10.' God's generosity could never be doubted by true Christians, asserted Hilder, but many feared that a large family would spell ruin.

> I have been the longer in this point, because distrust of the Lords providence in generall, (but more especially) relating to meanes for maintenance of many Children is growne to be an Epidemicall disease, overspreading the face of the Christian World.[7]

The same sorts of religious arguments against coitus interruptus were repeated by the herbalist physician Nicholas Culpeper:

That there is an Essential Vital Spirit in the Seed of both sexes, is without all question: (and that made up the basis of *Onan's* Sin mentioned in Scripture, in spilling his Seed; the other as circumstances did but aggravate it, for this God slew him. I beleeve God hath been more merciful to many in *England* in the same case, yet he is as just now as he was in *Onan's* day).[8]

By the eighteenth century the religious arguments in favour of large families were placing more and more emphasis on the practical benefits of such fecundity and, as far as Anglicans were concerned, the State accordingly had a duty to support the efforts of Christians to defend morality. The violation of the command to increase and multiply was, argued Richard Smalbroke, Bishop of St David's, an attack upon religious and civil society,

But as the Good of Society is the particular Care of the Magistrate, whatever has a direct Tendency to lessen the Number of Subjects, and to weaken or dishonour the Government, or bring it in to Confusion, falls under his immediate Cognizance.[9]

The arguments of Churchmen opposed to contraception had thus become to an extent secularized with mercantilist assumptions increasingly colouring their concerns.

Turning to those early writers who dealt with the subject of political economy one finds that the fears of overpopulation of the early seventeenth century were soon replaced with the classic mercantilist arguments, according to which increased population had to be pursued at all costs.[10] According to Hobbes:

Concerning multitude, it is the duty of them that are in sovereign authority to increase the people, in as much as they are governors of mankind under God Almighty, who having created but one man, and one woman, declared that it was his will they should be multiplied and increased afterwards. And seeing this is to be done by ordinances concerning copulation, they are by the law of nature bound to make such ordinances concerning the same, as may tend to the increase of mankind.[11]

It was the duty of state, according to such a premise, to 'forbid such copulations as are against the use of nature'. Hobbes's sentiments were echoed by John Graunt in his *Natural and Political Observations . . . Upon the Bills of Mortality* (1662) when expressing his outrage that 'such unlawfull Copulations beget Conceptions but to frustrate them by procured Abortions or secret Murthers'.[12] 'Populadia' in *A Discourse Concerning the Having Many Children* (1695) stated that such 'dishonourable embraces' resulted from the current fear of having large families. Men preferred to have barren wives out of a concern to live a life of ease. Only an heir was desired and after that no more children were wanted; parents would 'prescribe their number' and even pray against any more.[13]

Mercantilist and humanitarian concerns were linked up by those who, in the eighteenth century, campaigned in favour of establishing foundling homes. Addison, Cadogan, Coram and Hanway – presenting themselves as pro-natalists warring against the forces of depopulation – sought to protect both the born and unborn from their own parents. In Addison's *Guardian* of 11 July 1713 appeared a long defence of charitable institutions:

> But what Multitudes of Infants have been made away by those who brought them into the World, and were afterwards either ashamed or unable to provide for them!
>
> There is scarce an Assizes where some unhappy Wretch is not Executed for the Murder of a Child. And how many more of these Monsters of Inhumanity may we suppose to be wholly undiscovered, or cleared for want of Legal Evidence? Not to mention those, who by Unnatural Practices do in some Measure defeat the Intentions of Providence and destroy their Conceptions even before they see the Light. In all these the Guilt is equal, tho' the Punishment is not so. But to pass by the greatness of the Crime, (which is not to be expressed by Words) if we only consider it as it robs the Commonwealth of its full Number of Citizens, it certainly deserves the utmost Application and Wisdom of a People to prevent it.[14]

Addison's answer, as far as infanticide was concerned, was to establish the French-style foundling home or *tour* which allowed children to be secretly left in the care of authorities.

Such references to abortion and infanticide played a key role in the justification of a variety of eighteenth-century charitable institutions.[15] The anonymous promoter of a hospital for deserted children declared that poverty drove some poor women to prostitution:

> Sometimes these very Circumstances that I have mentioned, *prompt* the Mothers to much *worse Actions*, and put them upon Methods *to procure Abortions*, and, in case these should fail, to *destroy* their Infants *in their very Birth*, or *murder them* soon after.[16]

In *The Wisdom and Duty of Preserving Destitute Children* (1753) the Bishop of Worcester implied that even legitimate children were sometimes abandoned and so there was all the more reason to have institutions which could support the population growth of the country. In his estimation, numbers were declining

> not only in the Diminution of the present Generation, by *various* Methods of Destruction, and *numerous* Removals into other Countries; but also, when increasing *Lewdness* and fatal *Imtemperance* by spreading their baneful Influence . . . prevent the Increase of the next Generation.[17]

Jonas Hanway, in defining his charitable endeavours, argued that the ignorant and vicious poor had to be corrected, the bad parent punished and infants protected in order to promote population growth; and for the same reasons declared, 'such methods as *seem* to recommand a *promiscuous commerce*, must be shunned with great care, on *political* as well as *religious* principles'.[18]

That recourse to a variety of fertility-control methods was repeatedly attacked by sixteenth-, seventeenth- and eighteenth-century moralists has been noted. But the point being made here – that such protests and condemnations would not have been necessary if in fact such restriction of fertility was unthinkable – is often missed. There is also the issue of the implicit defences of contraception. In the first place, it was acknowledged by many that intercourse was indulged in primarily for the pleasure it gave, not for the child that might result. Culpeper, pro-natalist as he was, admitted that 'where the desire for children moves one to the act of copulation, the pleasure in the act moves a hundred'.[19] The compiler of the 1772 edition of *Aristotle's Masterpiece*, having examined the many ways in which births could be promoted, concluded the discussion with the insight: 'there are some that desire not to have

Children, and yet are very fond of nocturnal Embraces, to whom these Directions will be no way acceptable, because it may produce those Effects which they had rather be without'.[20] Author Reid began *The Pleasures of Matrimony* with the statement:

> I doubt but that it is an allay to many of one's nocturnal pleasures, to think upon the charge he is bringing upon himself, by satisfying a little amorous itch; but when he had done it and done it, and done it again, and finds there is no danger, then he falls to it without fear or wits. Besides there is another conveniency, they may live more plentifully, here are no portions to provide for children; when others are forced to sell part, and sometimes all their patrimony, to provide portions for their children.[21]

It has been noted by others that though Pepys never produced any children there is in his diary no expression of any great concern regarding this matter. To have a 'quiverful' of children was esteemed by many to be a great blessing but some felt no remorse at being spared such rewards.

The second argument advanced in favour of fertility control was that it was necessary in order to spare the woman a ceaseless series of pregnancies. Women who were judged to breed too quickly were warned by female friends and relatives to take the necessary measures to protect themselves. In 1749 Lady Mary Wortley Montagu wrote to her daughter,

> I don't know whether I shall make any court to you in saying it, but I own I can't help thinking that your family is numerous enough, and that the education and disposal of four daughters is employment for a whole life.[22]

One is reminded of the famous letters Madame de Sévigné addressed to her daughter in the 1670s. After the birth of a third grandchild Madame de Sévigné asked her daughter, 'What! douches [restringents] are not known in Provence?' and then cautioned her, 'I pray you, my dear, don't pride yourself on two beds; it is only a temptation; have someone sleep in your room'.[23]

The problem of providing dowries was advanced by seventeenth- and eighteenth-century writers as the third reason for limiting family size. In Charles Sedley's *Bellamira or, The Mistress* (1722) a character echoes Madame de Sévigné in declaring to his wife: 'we will have two Beds, for I will not come home Drunk and get Girls, without I knew where to get Portions for 'em; in this Age they sowre and grow stale upon their Parents hands'.[24] The Earl of Clarendon similarly referred to the alderman who 'was old before he married, and thought more of leaving his Children rich than of getting them, and so went warily to work'.[25] The anonymous writer of *Populousness with Oeconomy* (1769) complained: 'The many difficulties of providing for a numerous family are a discouragement to matrimony'.[26] For the poor, of course, it would be the problem of providing not dowries but simple food and clothing that could blunt the desire for a large family.

The fourth and most surprising argument against reproduction was that advanced by those who argued that children were often not worth the trouble of raising. This curious line of attack ran completely against the pro-natalist tide one associates with early modern England. William Whately in *A Care-Cloth or the Cumbers and Troubles of a Marriage* (1624) reviewed the difficulties of bearing children, their accidents and illnesses, and then the lewd and rebellious acts that such 'vipers' would inevitably be drawn to. According to William Ramsey, children were '*certain cares* and *uncertain comforts*'.[27] To back up his argument he drew up a list of infamous sons who had betrayed their fathers; every Jacob had his Levi, every David his Absalom, every Solomon his Rehoboam. These sorts of writings drew in part on the even older misogynist themes in literature that depicted marriage as a trap laid by women for men. The suspicion of children is a facet of the argument that has not received much attention. Perhaps its fullest expression was made in a work produced in 1673 by Samuel Dugard.

> Truly I have been sometimes apt to think that the want of an offspring has not been so great an unhappiness to some men, as commonly it is imagin'd to be. For what Father almost is there, who has not a greater vexation in his Children, than he would have in a Childless condition? . . . I might, Sir, Mention the great affliction that some men have from their Children when their Number increases, and they not withall to breed them up answerable to the Love they have for them, or that condition they themselves have alwaies liv'd in; a thing, which, I question not, had made some persons reflect upon their once joyfull wedding day with Care and Sorrow;

and wish they had either never known Marriage, or had been blest in a *Barren Womb*.[28]

One does not find in the early modern period an explicit defence of fertility control based on an acceptance of the married individual's right to remain purposefully childless. To marry was to become, or to anticipate becoming, a parent. But if some children were welcomed, not all were. In the literature there existed the clear expectation that out of concerns for the health of the mother and existing children, and for the well-being of the family as a whole, it would be understandable if in certain situations fertility were limited. The restriction of births was in early modern England thus thinkable; was it possible?

Some scholars believe that even if earlier generations wanted to limit their fertility they could not have succeeded because they lacked the necessary technology. Patricia James, the recent biographer of Malthus, writes 'Contraceptive practices could not become general until the vulcanization of rubber made possible the mass production of a variety of hygienic appliances'.[29] This statement is questionable, though, and in the following pages the wide range of techniques employed to limit fertility in the early modern period will be reviewed – restrictions on marriage and on coitus, post-partum taboos, extended lactation, observation of a woman's monthly cycle, employment of magical and herbal potions, recourse to coitus interruptus and use of various barrier methods – in order to show that, by means and for ends frequently foreign to the twentieth-century mind, control over births *was* sought in past times.

The first three factors that clearly affected fertility in early modern England were age of marriage, fecundity and frequency of coitus. We know most about the first factor and very little about the other two. The age of marriage of men had little impact on fertility rates, but the fact that English women did not normally marry before the age of twenty-five and entered menopause at about forty clearly restricted their potential childbearing years. In addition, many marriages were broken by the death of a spouse. Even assuming that a couple did enjoy fifteen years of marriage there was the possibility that sickness and poor diet would seriously undermine their sexual passions and their fecundity.[30] This in turn could adversely restrict the frequency of coitus. Tietze has estimated that in twentieth-century America, twenty-five to fifty acts of coitus are on average usually required for one conception. Given the presumed higher level of foetal wastage and stillbirths, and the lower level of fecundity in the seventeenth and eighteenth centuries, a lessening of coital frequency would have had all the greater negative effect on the birth rate.[31]

Typical English families of the early modern period were not, as a consequence, as large as is sometimes thought: the average number of children was between four and six. Long intervals of between twenty-four and thirty months separated each birth. Thus the 'birth control' employed by earlier generations resulted not in a concentration of births in the first years of marriage, as would be the case in the twentieth century, but in spacing births throughout the woman's fertile years and possibly in terminating them when she neared menopause. The fact that birth intervals became greater with age could be explained by declining fecundity, increased employment of methods of fertility restriction or a combination of the two.[32]

Turning from the social and physiological restrictions on fertility we can, for the purposes of this analysis, divide early modern English contraceptive behaviour into two categories – the negative, in which some type of abstinence from coitus was relied upon, and the positive, in which a strategy or device was employed to permit coitus to take place without conception ensuing.

The first type of abstinence was simple cessation of conjugal relationships during certain months of the year. In the previous chapter it was noted that the months of spring and early summer were considered the most fruitful and those of the late summer the least. Demographers have shown that seventeenth- and eighteenth-century birth rates did wax and wane as the year went on but why this should have been the case has not been fully explained.[33] Some have suggested that the traditional taboos against sex during Lent had a long life even in Protestant England. Others have argued that the fluctuations in births revealed a conscious attempt by a farming community to avoid having babies born in the early summer when labour was most required on the land. It should also be noted that the pious, who abstained during Lent, would presumably have done the same on Sundays and Saints' Days which would have appreciably lowered the frequency of coitus.

The second form of abstinence was the observance of the

post-partum taboo against intercourse while a mother was nursing. Lactation induces in a majority of women post-partum amenorrhoea, that is they do not ovulate and cannot conceive, but we are also told that for those women who do ovulate during nursing there is the chance that a subsequent conception will dry up their milk supply.[34] In an age when the only safe food for the child was mother's milk there would have been all the more reason for the woman to attempt to extend the nursing period as long as possible and to protect the milk supply by practising sexual abstinence. The likely fate of the child who was too quickly weaned was succinctly summed up in the seventeenth-century proverb, 'Soon todd [toothed] soon with God.'[35]

The practice of long nursings to space births was first seriously examined by medical doctors in the nineteenth century. In 1842 Dr Laycock reported that his investigations of women's childbearing histories at Manchester indicated that about 75 per cent of women did not conceive while lactating. On average, it was only two to three months after the weaning of one child that the next was conceived. As a result of both the nursing and the taboo against intercourse few mothers found themselves dealing with a rapid succession of births.[36] Many nineteenth-century observers noted that working-class women in particular clung to this strategy, extending their nursings to up to two years and beyond.[37] Alexander Milne, who was hostile to such attempts to limit family size, expressed his satisfaction that the method was not foolproof. He cited a popular ditty that held,

If women want from children to be freed,
To trust in nursing's but a broken reed.[38]

The very fact that such a song existed suggests that by the nineteenth century, at least, family limitation was pursued by extending the lactation period. What of the earlier period?

The desire to see mothers nursing their own offspring was repeatedly expressed in the early texts concerning childhood but its relationship to the spacing of births was not always recognized. The concern of most male writers was for the health of the child, not for the protection from pregnancy of the mother. Thus the Bishop of Exeter, having castigated those women who showed less maternal love than the tiger, wolf and bear, paraded his concern for the infant raised by a nurse:

Lastly, the dangers of this are not a few, if they were well considered. For manie a disease and ill qualitie is drawne with the milk from a bad nurse, besides that experience teacheth us, that manie plants will never prosper, except they have of their own earth about them.[39]

The 'Eminent Physician' who authored *The Nurse's Guide* (1729) added an eighteenth-century philosophical gloss on such sentiments:

The Duty of a Mother does not consist in conceiving, or bringing a Child into the World, but in bringing it up, and giving it all the Advantages of Education that can be imagined. A Mother conceives a Child from a Motive of Pleasure; She brings him into the World out of a natural Necessity; but the good Education she gives him, can proceed from nothing but good Will, Tenderness and Affection, which a Child can never sufficiently acknowledge.[40]

William Cadogan, John Nelson, George Armstrong and Michael Underwood all attacked those eighteenth-century women of fashion who handed over their children to mercenary nurses.[41] The campaign against such betrayals was capped in 1798 by the translation into English by William Roscoe of Luigi Tansillo's *The Nurse*. In melodramatic verse were charged those women who took the baby and 'To hireling hands its helpless frame convey'. In contrast to the pelican who used her own blood to nurse her young, Tansillo presented society women employing potions to terminate their lactating.

O crime! With herbs and drugs of essence high,
The sacred fountains of the breast to dry![42]

Judging by the comments of Archenholtz who was touring Britain in the late 1700s the campaign in favour of nursing did have some positive results:

Women of quality often suckle their own children, they do not consider the name nor the duties of a mother disgraceful, and they little value the loss of some charms in comparison with the sweets of maternal tenderness, and the agreeable consequences that result from them.[43]

What the men who campaigned for maternal nursing in the

eighteenth century chose to overlook was the fact that it was the husband who frequently prevented extended lactation. The reformers repeatedly criticized flighty females for failing to perform their maternal duty but failed to note that it could be countered by the husbands who demanded that their spouses fulfil their conjugal duty. It was a traditional belief that intercourse had to be avoided during nursing. In *The Art and Science of Preserving Bodie and Soul* (1579) John Jones cited Galen to the effect that venery could provoke menstruation, poison the milk, cause conception and dry up the breast by directing blood away from the paps to the womb.[44] Thus sexual desires had to be kept down by cold foods such as lettuce and water lilies. Turning from physiological to religious concerns, the Puritan William Gouge wrestled with the issue of whether the 'due benevolence' owed by spouses should be suspended while the woman nursed.

> *Quest.* What if the wife give sucke to her child, ought not her husband then to forbeare?
> *Answ.* Because giving sucke is a mother's duty, and hindered by breeding and bearing another child, man ought to doe what hee can to containe for that time: yet dare I not make this an inviolable law for man and wife to deny due benevolence each to other, all the time that the wife giveth sucke.[45]

That older post-partum taboos were being eroded was indicated by 'A.M.', author of *A Rich Closet of Physical Secrets* (1652), who asserted: 'Also copulation of the Nurse exceedingly offendeth, and hurteth the Child, as that which chiefly retraceth and diminisheth the Milk. . . . For which cause, in times past, Husbands were driven away from their Wives, and restrained from their companies'.[46] In referring to the fact that husbands had to be 'driven away' the anonymous writer was pointing out the fact that the desire of the woman to extend her nursing for the sake of herself and her child might run counter to the sexual desires of her mate.[47] The Earl of Clarendon raised the issue to the level of a possible threat to population when he suggested that,

> it would be a great Loss to the Commonwealth in lessening the Number of the People, if every Mother were obliged to nurse all the Children she brings forth; except you think that might be recompensed by the Number their Husbands would get in other Places whilst they are idle.[48]

On a more personal level the grand-niece of Lord John Cavendish found that her nursing a daughter raised the ire of her aristocratic relatives. What they wanted was a string of potential male heirs and as soon as possible. Such expectations were dashed by her nursing which postponed further conceptions. It was explained to the duchess that what made the family 'abuse suckling is their impatience for my having a son and their fancying I shan't so soon if I suckle'.[49]

Historical demographers investigating the impact of nursing have recently drawn attention to the fact that early modern England was remarkable in having both a very powerful force in highly variable nuptiality influencing total fertility but also in possessing quite low marital or completed fertility when compared to many other parts of Europe. Wrigley and Schofield and Wilson have shown that in general English villages throughout the seventeenth and eighteenth centuries were remarkable in having levels of marital fertility considerably lower than in large parts of Germany, France and the Low Countries. They argue that the evidence indicates that this difference cannot to any significant extent be accounted for by either primary or secondary sterility or differences in fecundability. By far the biggest influence, they conclude, was the degree of breastfeeding in the population. For instance, the village of Colyton studied by Wrigley had in the seventeenth and eighteenth centuries what demographers refer to as a 'mean post-partum nonsusceptibility period' of 13.7 months, that is 11.5 months greater than the 2.2 months of eighteenth-century Bavarian villages. In other words, the vast majority of English mothers in practising extended breastfeeding avoided the rapid succession of pregnancies suffered by their Bavarian counterparts who for some reason weaned their infants earlier. Lactation could, of course, only provide a woman with protection against a subsequent pregnancy for between six and twelve months; if sexual intercourse was resumed other methods of birth control would also have to have been employed to assure the extended birth interval of twenty-four to thirty months.[50]

The third form of abstinence that could affect fertility was restricting coitus to what was believed to be the sterile period in the woman's monthly cycle or what in the twentieth century has been called the rhythm method of birth control. Although the process of ovulation was not understood there existed from the time of the Greeks the conviction that the timing of menstruation was related to the timing of conception. The Galenic view held that menstrual blood was a surfeit that was discharged if a woman were not pregnant. If she had conceived her periods ceased because the blood was presumed to be turned to the purposes of nourishing the foetus.[51] Starting from such a premise it followed logically enough that doctors assumed that a conception would have the best chance of taking place immediately after a woman's period. Contrariwise, it was believed that the time just before a period would not be opportune because the 'flux' could wash away the seed.[52]

Most of the references we have to the woman's monthly cycle concerned ways in which to guarantee a fertile union. In 1656 Sadler, for example, wrote: 'The aptest time for conception is instantly after the months be ceast, because then the wombe is thirsty and dry, apt to draw the seed, and also to retaine it, by the roughnesse of the inward superficies'.[53] Nicholas Culpeper and John Pechey followed the same line of argument.[54] In the eighteenth century Willich explained that intercourse during a woman's period was necessarily infertile,

> besides which, the sexual intercourse during this period, as well as for some days immediately preceding, cannot answer the purpose of generation; because the ovum of the female, being but weakly attached is again separated by the periodic discharge. Hence the congress of the sexes is most generally crowned with fertility, after the catamenia have ceased; for then the female is in the most proper state for fecundation, so that the ovum has sufficient time to be consolidated, before the next menstrual evacuation.[55]

In the nineteenth century medical scientists continued to provide new evidence to support this old (but incorrect) schedule.[56]

Although the overt purpose of discussing the woman's cycle was to determine her most fertile period such analyses also inevitably discussed her least fertile. The condemnation made by moralists of intercourse during menstruation was based on their belief both in the woman's 'uncleanness' and in her inability to conceive. The Catholic Laurence Vaux condemned accordingly 'coming together at unseasonable times'.[57] The Puritan Perkins opposed intercourse 'so long as the woman is in her flowers' and his contemporary William Gouge attacked as an 'excess' such timing of sex.[58] The mercantilist William Petty grumbled, 'A man doth differ from all other animals in use of the female, and generation. By using the same without designe or desire of generation, and when generation is need-lesse or impossible'.[59]

Almost all of the references to the use of the cycle to restrict births were condemnatory. St Augustine lashed out at the Manichees for such practices.[60] In William Sermon's seventeenth-century work there was the implication, however, that such attempts were not all that blameworthy.

> Women are most subject to conceive a day, two, or three after their Courses be stopped, at which time they ought not (if they desire children) to use the act of Copulation too often, for that makes the womb too slippery, and more subject to open than to shut.[61]

Sermon was not openly defending a rhythm method of birth control but he allowed a glimpse of the attempts made by some to discover such a method.

Having dealt with the 'negative' forms of contraceptive behaviour that relied on some type of abstinence it is now possible to examine the 'positive' forms which permitted coitus without conception ensuing. Between the sixteenth and eighteenth centuries there were four main types of 'positive' contraception: by magic, by herbal potion, by coitus inter-ruptus and by appliance.

Just as magic was employed to elicit fertility so too was it used to guarantee barrenness. Some forms of magic were believed to have a long-term effect; others only affected each individual act of coition. The former would include, for example, the tradition in Bosnia of the new bride slipping her fingers under the groom's saddle.[62] She would, it was said, be barren for as many years as fingers she could squeeze in and free of children if both hands fitted. Similarly in Serbia if a dead child's coffin was nailed shut it implied that no other births were desired.[63] Such beliefs were reminiscent of the magical knots and locks employed in England. As suggested earlier in the discussion of ligatures (p. 40), it was believed that some women employed knots to impede their own fertility. Short-term magical contraception would include the use, reported by Le Roy Ladurie, by peasants in fourteenth-century France of amulets during intercourse to prevent pregnancies.[64] Albertus

Magnus gave instructions on the similar employment of the teeth of a child, the finger of a foetus and the testicles of a weasel.[65] The magical powers of the finger of a dead child were also noted by William Williams:

> The middle finger of an Abortive, being worn in a woman's neck, will keep her from conceiving. Jusquiammum mixed with the milk of a Mare, and laid upon a piece of Harts skin, and hung about a woman's neck keeps her from conceiving. If a woman takes a frog and opens his mouth, and spit in it thrice, she shall not conceive that year.[66]

Here again one finds examples of attempts at sympathetic magic. Just as the potions that rendered women barren were often drawn from 'fruitless' trees like the willow, many of the amulets implied that the woman was already with child and so unable to conceive. Spitting suggested the elimination of seed. Another range of potions employed menstrual blood with the presumed intent of aping the monthly cycle and so magically preventing conception.[67]

Herbal potions also had either long- or short-term contraceptive effects. For women who sought complete barrenness the writers of the herbals had a variety of suggestions.[68] In *The Garden of Health* Langham asserted that 'The flowers of a Sallow or Willow, maketh cold all heat of carnall lust' and 'causeth barrenness'.[69] In *Blagrave's Supplement of Enlargement to Mr. Nicholas Culpeper's English Physician* (1677) Guinny Pepper was said to have similar properties: 'if a piece of the Pod or husk, either green or dry be put into the Mother after delivery it will make them barren for ever after'.[70] The herbal writers recommended to men a variety of anti-aphrodisiac remedies to 'abate lust'. Some served as sorts of amulets such as the hemlock which Sowerby recommended wearing on the genitals.[71] Another author agreed that, 'Hemlockes bounde to a man stones, take utterly awaye all desyre of copulation'.[72] Of somewhat similar magical intent was Coles's suggestion that 'If a man gather *Vervaine* the first day of the New Moon, before Sun rising, and drinks the juyce thereof, it will make him avoid Lust for seven years'.[73] Langham likewise guaranteed that 'Leaves (of woodbine) drunk seven and thirtie days together, so dryeth up the naturall seede of man, that he shall gette no moe [sic] children'.[74] In general, the cooling plants and herbs were most praised for abating lust: *Agnus castus*, camphor, cannabis, dill, female fern, gourds, hemlock, honeysuckle, lettuce, lily, nenuphar, rue, spleenwort, tuftan and woodbine.[75] By following through the herbals the discussion of the efficacy of *Agnus castus* or the chaste tree one gets a notion of the decline in the belief in the power of such herbs. In sixteenth- and seventeenth-century herbals the chaste tree is said to extinguish the passions, but by 1722 Joseph Miller is writing that though once reputed to 'allay venereal Heats' *Agnus castus* is no longer employed; the *Compleat Herbal* of 1787 concludes, 'there is little use made of it now'.[76] These long-term contraceptive potions had as their main goal the bridling of the passions and were merely ways of reinforcing abstinence by herbal means.

For short-term contraceptive protection one could peruse the herbals for potions that would 'dry up seed' without adversely affecting lust. Such drugs were available. Langham reported that 'Rue eaten a certain space, drieth up natural seede in man', 'dill being drunk, it stoppeth the seede', hemp 'drieth up natural seede' and nenuphar 'in concoctions drunke, is good against Venus and fleshly lusts, or the same used in meates, or powder, doeth the like, and drieth up the seede of generation'.[77] Barrough stated that 'Purslaine eaten, and lettuce seede drunke, and the roote and seede of water Lillies taken in meate, do extinguish the seede by cooling of it. But Rew eaten corrupteth and destroyeth the seede with his heate'.[78] Lovell recommended that mint 'hindereth generation by condensating the sperme', Gerarde and Gesner praised honeysuckle and Cole added to the list spleenwort, colloquintada, wild cucumber, scammery, savin and hempstead.[79] The theory was that these herbs would dry up seed but not necessarily abate the passions. Coitus could thus take place without conception occurring.

A range of potions was specifically prescribed for women. Gerarde reported that poplar tree bark made women barren 'if drunk with the kidney of a mule after the flowers be ended'.[80] Frampton stated that sassafras caused barrenness by raising the heat of the womb.[81] Lovell noted the effects of aspern, ferne flagge, miltwast, mint, vetch and woodbine for similar purposes.[82] In the seventeenth century such remedies were mentioned with surprising nonchalance. In Ben Jonson's *Epicoene* two characters discuss these potions:

Epicoene: . . . and have you those excellent receipts, Madam, to keep from bearing children?
Haughty: O yes, Morose: how should we maintain our youth and beauty else?[83]

By the eighteenth century the literary portrayals of reliance on herbal contraceptives were adamantly hostile. Defoe presented in his *Treatise* a young bride asking a friend: 'there be Things to prevent Conception; an't there?' She does consume some drug and for two years has no children, but her husband grows suspicious. 'Her Apprehensions now were, that Her Husband should suppose either that she still used Art with her self to prevent her being with Child, or to destroy a Conception after it had taken place'. Fearing that he might have the marriage annulled the wife begs the husband's forgiveness and

> assured him of her being fully satisfied that it was unlawful, and that she had committed a great Crime in what she had done before; that it was a Sin against her Husband; that she had injured him in it, dishonoured her self, and offended against the Laws both of God and Man'.[84]

Did these early 'oral contraceptives' work? One presumes that most did not have the desired physiological effect but it is possible that some were successful. Reporting on the use of similar plant materials by a wide variety of 'primitive groups' in the twentieth century Nag warned:

> The efficacy of these contraceptive drugs cannot, however, be totally dismissed. It is well known that some plants contain substances, such as steroids, enzymes, and hormonal agents, that affect the reproductive process in animals and human beings. . . . The available literature does not, however, assist in learning the possible efficacy of the drugs used by the societies in my selection.[85]

The third major form of 'positive' contraception was the employment of coitus interruptus or whatever position might best frustrate conception. By the nineteenth century the withdrawal method of birth control had become the main brake on fertility. How widely the practice was employed in the early modern period is difficult to judge. It is also unclear whether it was a method that had to be 'taught' or if each couple could

discover it for themselves. Perhaps the earliest English reference to the practice comes in John of Gaddesden's (1280–1336)
The English Rose in which women were warned of the sinful-
ness of 'jumping backwards or too sudden a motion after
coitus'.[86] In the sixteenth century Dr Layton, reporting to
Cromwell on the debaucheries of the Abbey of St Mary at York,
wrote that the clergy were involved, 'in kyndes of knaverie, as,
*retrahere membrum virile in ipso punctu seminis emittendi, ne inde
fieret prolis generatio*, and nunnes to take potations *ad prolem
conceptum opprimendum*'.[87] The method of withdrawal was
known in the early modern period as Onanism. Onan,
according to the book of Genesis, had defied God's command to
have children by his dead brother's wife and cast his seed
upon the ground for which he was punished by death. Whether
God slew Onan simply because of his defiance or because of the
specific form it took was never made clear. In the main,
however, it was the contraceptive aspects of the act that
preoccupied moralists. Thus Babington warned in a 1596 text:
'And concerning the fact of Onan thinke no better of it, than
you do that a woman should destroy her fruitfulness, for this in
a man is even that sinne: an uglie, foule & filthie wickednes'.[88]
The Puritan Gouge informed his readers that they would be as
guilty as Onan should they follow his example: 'It is so much
the more heinous when hatred, stoutnesse, nicenesse, fear of
having too many children, or any other like respects, are the
cause thereof'.[89] Even a seventeenth-century wife complained,

> that her husband did not deal with her in bed as befitted a
> married man, nor as other women were dealt withall by their
> husbands, for that he carnally coupled with her of late years
> but once a quarter and then what seed should be sowen in the
> right ground he spent about the outward part of her body and
> withall threatened if she were with child he would slit the gut
> out of her belly.[90]

But the fact that a variety of euphemisms were employed to
describe the practice gives some support to the argument that
this method of contraception was not considered by many to be
all that outrageous. In Grose's *A Classical Dictionary of the
Vulgar Tongue* under the heading COFFEE HOUSE followed the
explanation 'to make a coffee house of a woman's ****, to go in
and out and spend nothing'.[91] More common were aphorisms
based on agrarian analogies. Guillemeau explained a woman's

barrenness as being a result of 'her husband having never entered within her maiden cloister: and that with threshing onely at the barn doore, she could not be full'.[92] de Brantôme referred to another who 'would even grind at his ladies mill', and an older London woman advised a pregnant woman as how not to get in 'that way' again with the words 'You must leave it at the mill door'.[93]

Beginning in the early eighteenth century there were some, however, who sought to exploit for commercial ends the fear that sexual excesses could result from either masturbation or coitus interruptus. The fact that both practices were referred to as onanism permitted quacks to compound both moral and medical arguments in asserting that the wasting of seed led to physical debilitation.

Having terrified their readers with a long list of illnesses that could be caused by onanism – debility, consumption and loss of hearing, memory and eyesight – quacks sought to lure the frightened into a purchase of some restorative. For example, in the early editions of *Onania* Thomas Crouch advertised his 'Strengthening Tincture' and 'Prolific Powder'. In the 1730 edition it was announced that Crouch had died and that J. Isted would now supply the necessary cordials and draughts. As the century wore on more and more remarkable remedies appeared. W. Farrer brought out a 'Restorative Nervous Elixir', W. Brodum sold a 'nervous Cordial and Botanical Syrup', E. Senate advertised 'Steel Lozenges', James Graham lauded the benefits of an 'Elixir of Life', and Samuel Solomon boasted of the vast sale of his 'Cordial Balm of Gilead'.[94]

The first English work on the subject was an anonymous text entitled *Of the Crime of Onan . . . or the Heinous Vice of Self-Defilement* and from the first page set out to terrify and titillate the reader. The first edition, which appeared sometime before 1717, confined itself primarily to describing the horrible fate that awaited those given to masturbation or what was called the 'school-wickedness'. The author conceded that some would find his work shocking but declared that it was far better that youth be warned than face the eventual judgement of God.

The great Account Book then shall lie
Open to every Offender's Eye,
To try his Self-Defilements by.
   Then sits the Judge upon his Throne,

And makes all Self-Defilement known,
When each Onanian knows HIS OWN.[95]

But the warnings were not restricted to the private vices of youth; passing reference was also made to 'The Use, Abuse of, and Frustrating the Marriage Bed' which implied that more than mere masturbation was being condemned. This line of argument was followed up in a work of 1724 entitled *Eronia: On the Use and Abuse of the Marriage Bed by Er and Onan*. Here the reader was reminded that Er had sinned because, out of a desire to maintain his wife's beauty, he had sought to free her from the burden of childbearing. The author then went on to censure those married persons who indulged in 'Embraces that may be thought *Frustraneous*, because Procreation may not be at that Time attainable'.

There are some Married Persons in the World who think Children come too fast, and distrusting the Capacity of maintaining them, frustrate what is appointed for the *Continuance of our Species*. This is a Frustraneous Abuse of the Marriage-Bed, and a very great Crime, which every one ought to avoid, and submit to *Providence* for the Maintenance of what determinate *Number of Children* it has allotted for them.[96]

It is of interest to note that the author assumed that only members of the upper classes engaged in such vices because he called on his audience to remember that 'Working and Labouring People', although only living from hand to mouth, made no attempt to limit their fertility.

The fourth edition of *Onania* contained a letter from a woman who declared that the sole purpose of marriage was procreation and that therefore any sexual activity that did not result in offspring was sinful. The author gave the impression that he agreed with her judgement and directly attacked husbands who adopted a strategy which he dubbed the 'retreat'.

Thousands there are in the married State who provoke and gratify their Lust, as far as is consistent with their destructive Purpose, and no farther, which being as I have said before a Sin of a deep Die, it is hoped, by what is here said of it they will in Time take warning and Repent of.[97]

In the seventh edition of *Onania*, dated 1723, the author changed tack and in reply to the same letter declared that marriage was not simply established for procreation; conjugal amity was as important. But having said this he returned to the attack on the use of coitus interruptus as a means of birth control:

> there are Married persons, who commit a heinous Sin to God, by frustrating what he has appointed for the Multiplication of our Species, and are commonly such, as think Children come too fast, and distrust Providence for their Maintenance and Education. They indulge themselves in all the Pleasures of the Sense, and yet would avoid the Charges they might occasion; in order to which they do what they can to hinder Conception. What I mean, is, when the Man, by a criminal untimely Retreat, disappoints his Wife's as well as his own fertility. This is what may be call'd a frustraneous Abuse of their bodies and must be an abominable Sin. Yet it is certain, that Thousands there are in the Married State, who provoke and gratify their Lust, as far as is consistent with the destructive Purpose, and no further.[98]

What is remarkable about the fifth and seventh editions of *Onania* is that in addition to the condemnations of onanism they also included a letter which appears to be the earliest defence of the withdrawal method of birth control. The writer identified himself as a poor man with three children, who, because of poverty, had to agree with his wife to limit the size of their family.

> Now Sir, this melancholy View, which might be much more aggravated, drove us by consent upon this expedient you generally and justly condemn in your Answer to the Ladies [sic] Letter: My conscience seem to Clear me of ONAN's crime, for what he did was out of spite and ill will, and contrary to an express Command of raising up Seed to his Brother, in Contradiction to the Method of our Redemption: Whereas mine is pure necessity in respect both of Body and Soul.[99]

The author printed this plea but did not agree with the sentiments expressed. He charged the writer with lack of faith and failure to recognize the physical dangers of his deed. Now it is possible, indeed probable, that the letter was manufactured by the author as an expository device but even if this were the case it still follows that the argument it contains – namely

79

that coitus interruptus was morally justifiable – was presumed by him to be held by many of his prospective readers.

The suggestion that couples were seeking to control fertility by assuming various coital positions was also made in the oldest and most widely read sex manual of the time, *Aristotle's Masterpiece*.[100] In the 1772 edition there was reference made to couples who did not want children: 'there are some that desire not to have children and yet are very fond of nocturnal Embraces'.[101] The tactics such couples might adopt is suggested by what the manual condemns. Thus the anonymous author warns husbands not to withdraw too quickly for to do so permits cold air to strike the womb and cause illness. Women are cautioned to lie still after coition and in particular to refrain from sneezing. Sneezing at the crucial moment was to enjoy a long reputation as an effective defensive tactic.

The eighteenth-century reader could find similarly helpful information by perusing *Conjugal Love Reveal'd; in the Nightly Pleasure of the Marriage BED and the Advantages of that Happy STATE in an Essay Concerning Human Generation Done from the French of Monsieur Venette*. Here, as in *Aristotle's Masterpiece*, one would read, 'Nature has taught both Sexes such Positions as are allowable, and that contribute to Generation; and Experience has shown those that are forbidden and contrary to Health.' Couples were warned that to take up such non-prolific positions led to the harming of any possible offspring.[102] Much the same argument was made by John Armstrong who, in the *Oeconomy of Love: A Poetical Essay*, called on his countrymen to refrain from embraces which, being unnatural, had to be of foreign origin:

> But in these vicious Days great Nature's Laws
> Are spurned; eternal Virtue, which nor Time,
> Nor Place can change, nor Custom changing all,
> Is mocked to scorn; and lewd Abuse instead,
> Daughter of the Night, her shameless Revels holds
> O'er half the Globe, which the chaste face of Day
> Eclipses at her Rites. For Man with Man,
> And Man with Woman (monstrous to relate!)
> Leaving the natural Road, themselves debase
> With Deeds unseemly, and Dishonour foul.
> Britons, for shame! Be Male and Female still.
> Banish this foreign Vice; it grows not here,

It dies neglected; and in Clime so chaste
Cannot but by forc'd Cultivation thrive.[103]

It is worth noting, that in the literature dealing with coital
positions the idea of the 'woman on top' was invariably condemned. On the one hand this reflected the traditional male
view that the woman had to be both literally and figuratively
'under' men.[104] On the other hand there is evidence to suggest
that the fear of the woman being on top was also motivated by
the belief that in assuming such a position she could avoid
pregnancy. In the popular poem 'Kick Him Jenny' appeared the
lines:

Thus in a Chair the cautious Dame,
Who loves a little of the Same,
Will take it on her Lover's Lap,
Sure to prevent, this way, Misshap:
Subtle Lechers! Knowing that,
They cannot so be got with Brat.[105]

The information that can be gleaned from the texts on couples'
adoption of coitus interruptus or positions which were
believed to be inapt for conception is important for two
reasons. First, the references usually concern married people
and thus the practices were distinct from those associated with
prostitutes and their clients. Second, such practices required
the active participation of both partners; the woman was not
passive – indeed some have suggested that increased reliance
on coitus interruptus signified the success of females in
'domesticating' males.[106]

The fourth major form of 'positive contraception' was the one
with which twentieth-century readers would be most familiar –
the barrier method by which either the man or woman
employed some device that prevented the meeting of egg and
sperm. For the earlier period most of the references to such
practices assumed that the initiative would be taken by the
woman. There are recipes in sixteenth-century texts for
pessaries of rue and ground lily root combined with
castoreum.[107] In the seventeenth century James Ferrand
suggested a douche of castor oil and rue.[108] Leonard Sowerby
provided an extensive list of such recipes. He recommended a
pepper douche, 'Hatchet Fitch used as a suppository before the
carnal knowledge of man', and 'Mint applyed on the natural

place of women, before they knew men carnally'.[109] The purported effectiveness of these stratagems was that they lowered the heat of reproductive organs and so impeded conception. Today it would be surmised that their effectiveness would be directly related to their ability to immobilize the spermatozoa.

Turning to male contraceptive measures we come to a real innovation – the condom. Because of its ultimate importance as a contraceptive device many books on the history of birth control begin with a discussion of the sheath.[110] In a study of traditional methods of fertility control it is a moot point, however, as to how much attention should be paid to it. This is not because it was a 'modern' device nor because its expense limited its use to the upper classes until the end of the nineteenth century. The objection to including the condom in a discussion of early modern birth control is based rather on the fact that it was originally designed, not to prevent pregnancy, but to protect the male from venereal disease.

The first known printed description appeared in a passage dealing with syphilis in Gabriello Fallopio's posthumously published *De morbo gallico* (1564).[111] The earliest English reference seems to have been in John Marten's *A Treatise of all the Degrees and Symptoms of the Venereal Disease in Both Sexes* (1704). Marten cited Fallopio and the instrument Marten described was, like the earlier writer's, made of 'Lint or Linnen Rags' which were to be soaked in a special wash before engagement.[112] Marten refused to give details because of his avowed concern that if they became common knowledge sin would abound; his real intent, of course, was to draw customers to purchase his special anti-venereal solution.

Marten was not allowed to sell his instruments in peace. In 1711 a rival quack, J. Spinke, attacked him in a publication entitled *Venus's Botcher or, the Seventh Edition of Mr. Martin's* [sic] *(comical) Treatise of the Venereal Disease.*[113] It was Spinke's complaint that Marten by both advertising and disparaging the work of other practitioners was attempting to monopolize the market. Spinke stated that he had been singled out by Marten for special censure because he (Spinke) had done the greatest good with what he called the 'blue Apron' – presumably some rival form of prophylactic.

The sheaths were advertised in the same sorts of publications in which quacks paraded the benefits of their pills and potions.

That papers should carry such announcements raised the particular ire of Joseph Cam. In *A Rational and Useful Account of the Venereal Disease* (1737) he upbraided one promoter as being as guilty as the inventor:

> Surely, Sir, you advise all Mankind, which is prompt enough of itself to offend, to use *Machinery*, and to fight in *Armour*. If so, you are not the Inventor, but the *Propagator* of Wickedness: But we see how some Persons aim to deceive the world.[114]

In the eyes of Cam and respectable physicians the danger of 'preventives' was that they permitted the promiscuous to indulge their passions without fear of punishment. Indeed there were a number of eighteenth-century medical men who believed that even cures for venereal disease should, for the same reason, not be sought. For this reason it was assumed by many that doctors were chiefly opposed to the use of 'armour' because they feared the loss of much of their clientele. As early as 1709 this view was expressed in the *Tatler* which inaccurately reported that the philanthropic inventor of the sheath was a patron of Will's Coffee House:

> Such a Benefactor is a Gentleman of this House, who is observ'd by the Surgeons with much Envy; for he has invented an Engine for the Prevention of Harms by Love-Adventures, and has, by great Care and Application made it an immodesty to name his name.[115]

For some reason, which historians have not yet resolved, the name of this invention was associated in Englishmen's minds, not with John Marten, but with the apparently mythical Mr Condum. In Francis Grose's *A Classical Dictionary of the Vulgar Tongue* there appeared the citation: 'CUNDUM. The dried gut of a sheep, worn by men in the act of coition, to prevent venereal infection; said to have been invented by one colonel Cundum.' Interestingly enough the French also attributed the invention to the English. In *A Treatise of the Venereal Disease* Jean Astruc wrote:

> I am informed, that of late years the Debauchees in *England*, that set no bounds to their meretricious armours, make use of a little bag, made of a thin bladder, which they call a *condum*,

with this they arm the *penis*, that they may be preserved safe from the dangers of an engagement whose consequences are always doubtful. For they imagine, that being arm'd thus *cap-a-pe*, they may with great safety face the dangers of promiscuous venery.[116]

Astruc assured his readers that there was no way of avoiding the pox if it was not by leading a pure, chaste life. For the promiscuous to seek safety in a slim sheath he found laughable; in his opinion

they ought to arm their penis with oak, guarded with a triple plate of brass, instead of trusting to a thin bladder, who are fond of committing a part so capable of receiving infection to the filthy gulph of a Harlot.[117]

The sort of covering which Astruc envisaged clearly required a sacrifice of comfort in favour of security. Even the mid-eighteenth-century sheaths which were made of animal bladders or fine covering, tied at the open end with a ribbon, were not entirely satisfactory. They were too expensive to be used except by the wealthy and, because of the material of which they were made, required moistening before use; 'dipped my machine in the Canal and performed most manfully' wrote Boswell of one out-of-doors encounter.[118] Some found such inconveniences too much to bear. Daniel Turner in *Syphilis: A Practical Dissertation on the Venereal Disease* (1717) stated:

The *Condum* being the best, if not the only Preservative our Libertines have found at present; and yet, by reason of its blunting the Sensation, I have heard some of them acknowledge, that they had often to choose to risk a *Clap*, rather than engage *cum Hastis sic clypeatis* [with spears thus sheathed].[119]

Boswell was a case in point. He prided himself on engaging only when 'safely sheathed' or in 'armourial guise' but admitted that at times 'I found but a dull satisfaction'. On occasion he would chance an unencumbered encounter. He wrote of the night of 17 May 1763:

I picked up a fresh, agreeable young girl called Alice Gibbs. We went down a lane to a snug place, and I took out my armour, but she begged that I might not put it on, as the sport was much pleasanter without it, and as she was quite safe.[120]

As the passage from Boswell indicated women were not uninterested in the advantages and disadvantages of 'armour'. On occasion the prostitute provided her customer with the instrument. In his entry for 25 November 1762 Boswell wrote: 'I picked up a girl in the Strand; went into a court with intention to enjoy her in armour. But she had none'.[121] Indeed the two most famous retailers of these devices in the eighteenth century were women – Mrs Philips and Mrs Perkins. Grose cited an advertisement from the *St James Chronicle* in which Mrs Philips boasted of thirty-five years of experience 'in the business of making and selling machines, commonly called implements of safety, which serve the health of her customers'. The advertisement ended with the doggerel rhyme:

To guard yourself from shame or fear
Votaries to Venus, hasten here:
None in my wares e'er found a flaw
Self preservation's nature's law.

Mrs Perkins contented herself with informing the public in simple prose that at the Green Canister in Half-Moon Street opposite the New Exchange in the Strand she made and sold 'all sorts of fine machines, otherwise called C-MS'.[122]

Almost all the eighteenth-century references to sheaths concern their use by a man when consorting with a prostitute. The association of this instrument with vice would be a major reason why the respectable would long refuse to acknowledge its efficacy in controlling fertility. Yet even in the eighteenth century one can find the argument expressed that honourable women could use it to guard themselves from 'shame or fear'. Such seems to be the message of Joseph Gay's *The Petticoat: An Heroi-Comical Poem* published in 1716.

The NEW MACHINE a sure Defence shall prove,
And guard the Sex against the Harms of Love.

So might the Fair, thus arm'd remain secure
And brave the Dangers which they shun'd before,
Safe in their Ramparts all Assaults defie
And dare the Efforts of the Enemy.

Should now Good natur'd Nymphs (which Heav'n forfend!)
To grant too early favours condescend;
See here, the happy means propos'd to shun,
The fatal Danger, when the fault is done.[123]

The same argument was made more forcibly still in yet another poem, White Kennett's *The Machine or, Love's Preservative* (1724).

> Hear and attend: In CUNDUM's praise
> I sing and thou, O Venus! aid my Lays
>
> By this Machine secure, the willing Maid
> Can taste Love's Joys, nor is she more afraid
> Her Swelling Belly should, or squalling Brat,
> Betray the luscious Pastime she has been at.[124]

The sheath, the discussion of which enjoys the pride of place in so many histories of birth control, warrants no further discussion in this study. Despite its presumed greater effectiveness in preventing conception it could not – because of its cost and associations with prostitution – play any significant role in the rituals of reproduction which are the main concern of this work.[125]

In the 'primitive' societies investigated by anthropologists in the early twentieth century the same sorts of contraceptive measures employed by early modern English men and women – post-partum taboos, magic, coitus interruptus, douches and drugs to induce temporary or permanent sterility – were also found. But since such societies valued fertility so highly why were such practices employed? It was not necessarily to limit drastically the size of the family but often to allow the woman to avoid conception during the post-partum period when her first concern was to nurse the baby she already had. Though initially surprised by discovering the extent of the discussion of fertility-controlling strategies in England in the sixteenth, seventeenth and eighteenth centuries one slowly realizes that whatever legitimation contraception enjoyed was due to the fact that it must have been considered by some as simply a way of freeing a woman: not from pregnancy *per se*, but from too rapid a succession of pregnancies. If the taboo against post-partum sexual intercourse had been completely respected the spacing of children in the family could have been accomplished without such expedients. If the taboo was broken but its purpose – protection of the mother and existing child – was still to be sought, then recourse to some contraceptive strategy was called for. By the same logic, contraceptive measures were frequently employed in premarital and extramarital affairs to prevent births at the *wrong* time.

In reviewing the variety of contraceptive strategies available to past generations this chapter has sought to demonstrate that conscious restriction of fertility in early modern England was not only 'thinkable' but possible: the contemporary literature lends support to the argument that it was not any technological or moral revolution but new social pressures that underlay the dramatic decline in nineteenth-century fertility. One other form of fertility control – abortion – which was employed in pre-industrial England and has to be included in any account of family limitations is the subject of the following chapter.

4
'All manner of art, to the help of drugs and physicians': abortion as birth control

Emmenagogues are extensively used [in Buru] to avoid having children and, likewise artificial abortion is generally tolerated and often performed upon girls and women. The secret means used for this purpose do not seem to cause the body of the woman any lasting damage.
George Devereux, *A Study of Abortion in Primitive Societies* (1955)

In the early modern period most of the discussions of fertility control assumed that the woman bore the responsibility of spacing births. A Virginia mother wrote of her daughter in 1791: 'I cou'd wishe she did not have 'em quite so fast'. Catherine Vanhorne Read warned her pregnant sister at about the same time: 'I do not wish you to fill your nursery too soon'. Abigail Adams went so far as to welcome the news of the miscarriage of a relative saying 'it is sad slavery to have children as fast as she has'.[1] Men seemed strangely marginal in such discussions. Women were, of course, harder hit by a pregnancy whether it was desired or not and it followed that their attitudes towards family limitation would necessarily be distinct from those of their husbands. This issue has often been overlooked when the focus has been mainly on one means of fertility control – contraception. There is sometimes an assumption that the decline in fertility in the nineteenth century was a consequence of a diffusion of new knowledge and concentration on the role of mechanical contraceptives. But perhaps the major form of family limitation in past times was abortion. At a time when all the various forms of contraception

89

were lacking in reliability numerous women would have inevitably discovered that a 'mistake' had been made. What then? Clearly those intent on limiting births would have to contemplate the option of abortion as a second line of defence.

When we turn to an analysis of the role played by abortion in fertility control we are provided with a good example of how cultural anthropology can assist historical research. The study of abortion promises to cast a fresh light on a number of vital questions: women's responses to their reproductive function, male and female attitudes towards sexuality, and medical and moral concerns for embryonic life. The problem is that we know very little of the extent of the practice. Only after 1803 when abortion was made a statutory offence is it feasible to accumulate 'hard' evidence, not of all who had recourse to the practice, but at least of those who were unlucky enough to come to the attention of the authorities.[2] The fact that the pre-1803 period does not offer even these slim statistical sources has been a lacuna in largely quantitative analyses of family structure and attitudes determining it. But the hopes and fears, desires and delusions that escape statistical analysis are crucial for our understanding of attitudes towards reproduction, and only by examining ideas concerning abortion can one gain access to a separate culture – a world of female reproductive rituals – that has remained largely hidden. In this chapter we will attempt to determine who aborted, their motives, their helpers, their methods, their timing and their attitudes towards such practices.

Who sought to induce their own miscarriages in early modern England? Most of the reports we have attributed abortion to the unmarried – single and widowed women who sought to avoid an illegitimate birth. In 1590 the Vicar of Weaverham in Cheshire was denounced as 'an instructor of young folks how to commit the sin of adultery or fornication and not beget or bring forth children'.[3] In *The Expert Midwife* (1637) James Rueff asked rhetorically:

> For how many Virgins, how many Widdowes also ensnared and intangled with these Arts and divellish practices, have committed cruell and more than brutish murders of their tender Babes and Infants? When first being deflowered (and robbed of their best Jewell) they have perceived some alterations to be caused in them, as variable appetites, a loathing

of their accustomed meate and drinke, continuall vomiting, dispositions to parbrake in the morning, passions and pains of the heart, swoonings, paines of the teeth: by and by instructed with evil Arts, they make the first experiments by lacing in themselves strait and hard, that they may extinguish and destroy the feature conceived in their wombe. But when they receive no help thereby, they assay and attempt greater matters.[4]

'Help' might actually be forced upon the woman, as was the case reported in Maryland in 1652:

Susanna Warren testified that when Captain Mitchell perceived 'she bred Child by Him', he prepared a 'potion of Phisick', put it in an egg, and forced her to take it, and that two or three days afterward he had told her that if she were with child 'he would warrant that he had frighted it away.[5]

In seventeenth-century Somerset, Geoffrey Quaife uncovered numerous accounts of young women seeking to terminate a pregnancy after having been seduced by a master, fellow servant or in-law. Here too it was often the man who suggested recourse to some herbal cure. One, the court reported, 'did advise and press her [his mistress] to take bears-foot and savon boiled, and drink it in milk, and likewise, hay madder chopt, and boiled in beer and drink it to destroy the child conceived in this examinant's body'.[6] In the early eighteenth century Daniel Defoe was claiming that it was not infanticide alone that limited population growth: 'add to this procur'd Abortion and other indirect means, which wicked Wretches make use to screen themselves from the censure of the World, which they dread more than the Displeasure of their Maker'.[7]

The most common image of the woman seeking recourse to abortion was thus that of the single, lower-class female, usually a domestic. Miss Weeton wrote to a friend in 1807 of a kitchen maid:

Mary Downall is in a poor state of health. Mrs. Billington thinks her in a decline. I am afraid she took something when pregnant of her little girl intended to fall on the child, and it has light on herself. She has looked a bad colour ever since.[8]

Because abortion was associated with seduction it is not surprising to find that it attracted the attention of balladeers and novelists. The ancient folksong, 'Mary Hamilton', told the tale of a lover seeking an abortifacient for his lady.

> The king is to the Abbey gane,
>   To pu the Abbey-tree,
> To scale the babe frae Marie's heart,
>   But the thing it wadna be.[9]

In a second version it was the maiden who went to the 'deceivin' tree' which appeared to be a corruption for 'savin', a popular abortifacient. In yet another version collected by Sir Walter Scott the woman sang,

> My love he was a pottinger [apothecary]
>   Money drink he gave to me,
> And a'to put back that bonnie babe,
>   But alas, it wad na do.[10]

'Tam Lin' contained a similar theme of the man asking the woman:

> Why pu's thou the rose Janet,
>   Amang the groves sae green,
> And a'to kill the bonnie babe
>   That we gat us between.[11]

The theme of the seduced young girl forced to take an abortifacient by the man responsible for her condition also attracted the attention of women writers preoccupied by the inequities of the double standard. In *The Wrongs of Woman, or Maria: a Fragment* (1798) Mary Wollstonecraft presented the classic story of the servant girl whose seduction was followed, on the insistence of her master, by an abortion. 'After some weeks of deliberation had elapsed, I in continual fear that my altered shape would be noticed, my master gave me a medicine in a phial, which he desired me to take, telling me, without any circumlocution, for what purpose it was designed'.[12] Wollstonecraft's heroine survived her ordeal with remarkably little discomfort. A more frightening tale was told by the religious enthusiast Joanna Southcott in her *Letters and Communications . . . lately written to Jane Towley* (1804); here the seducer provided an abortifacient which killed both mother and child.

> And now the Truth thou must declare,
>   And tell the Woman's doom –

Now she with child, by him beguil'd,
And then the shame to Miss;
He brought the poison then for her,
But I shall answer this –
Savine you know is an herb doth grow
And there the poison laid;
He said the Child's life it would take
And there she was betray'd;
Because her own, he told her then,
Her life could never hurt;
'Twas but the child that would be slain,
Her honour to support.[13]

This stress on the recourse to abortion of abandoned single women seeking to avoid illegitimate births was based on the assumption of commentators that since induction of miscarriage was dangerous, the risk would deter all but the most desperate. Thomas Short, for example, referred to it as a form of 'suicide'.

If Whoredom be a fault, Suicide is a far greater Crime: by Suicide is meaned, not only the Destruction of real Beings in the Womb, Birth, or immediately after; but all nefarious Practices used by wicked Wretches to prevent Conception from their Carnal Gratification.[14]

Alexander Hamilton spoke in equally dark terms:

Some unfortunate women, to conceal their criminal indulgences, endeavour, by various means, to procure the expulsion of the child before it has acquired such a size that the situation can be discovered. . . . Whenever, therefore women commit such unjustifiable crimes to conceal the indulgence of irregular passions, their life is exposed to the greatest danger.[15]

Similar warnings were sounded by the anonymous author of *Thoughts on the Means of Alleviating the Miseries Attendant Upon Common Prostitution* (1799).

It is not possible to calculate the numbers who, thus circumstanced in mind and body, greedily accept and swallow the medicines in vulgar repute for procuring abortion. The ignorant administrators of these baleful drugs destroy the mother, perhaps, not less frequently than the embryo. This hazard, though often foreseen, is willingly encountered.[16]

93

And in case this barrage of moral injunctions was not heard Martha Mears, in *The Pupil of Nature: or Candid Advice to the Fair Sex* (1797), directly addressed women.

> My blood runs cold, and my hand trembles, in proceeding to describe the far more inevitable dangers that attend abortion brought on by artificial means. Ah! what a struggle between the emotions of pity for the sufferer, and of horror at the fatal cause! So wicked an outrage upon nature is sure to be punished with tortures and with death.[17]

The problem posed by the testimony left by the preceding authors is that they presented abortion in a lurid but simplistic fashion. They presented only one sort of woman – the seduced victim – and only one sort of motive – the desire to avoid an illegitimate birth. The fact that abortion was dangerous would, it was thought, limit its practice to the desperate. Since most of the women whose miscarriages came to the attention of the authorities were single, the argument that the practice was the last resort of the unmarried seemed to be confirmed. Upon closer investigation, however, it becomes clear why similar attempts by married women would go undetected. A married woman who miscarried raised few suspicions; with a single woman the chance existed that a master, father or neighbour would discover her condition and demand some explanation. Moreover, in a time of trouble a single woman would have fewer resources at her disposal, she would have fewer people to whom she could turn and the likelihood of discovery was therefore all the greater. The married woman, sooner recognizing the first signs of pregnancy, could respond more quickly and effectively to the situation; the single, perhaps hoping that a speedy marriage would obviate the necessity of an abortion, might well postpone action until it was too late.

But why would married women for whom an unexpected pregnancy did not necessarily entail – as it did for the single – social ostracism and poverty have recourse to abortion? The desire to control their own fertility provided the first reason. A careful sifting of the evidence allows one to catch glimpses of serious and determined women who appreciated the dangers of the practice but regarded it as their right, should the needs of their health and the well-being of their families so demand. Each and every pregnancy was not welcomed by the married. Mrs Alice Thornton, on discovering her pregnancy in 1667, confided to her diary 'if it had been good in the eyes of my God, I should much rather . . . not have been in this condition'. If abortion was frightening so too were 'the Dangers and Pains of a hard Travail, weakness of Constitution, hereditary Miscarriages and such like'.[18] Married women so encumbered who sought to induce miscarriage could be assisted by their husbands: the 'subtle persons' referred to by Pechey 'who shall tell you fine stories of the diseases of the Wives'.[19] Lady Caroline Fox, finding herself pregnant for the third time in almost as many years, wrote her husband 'I'm certainly breeding, I took a great deal of physic yesterday in hopes to send it away, but it has only convinced me my fears prove true'. Shortly thereafter she found that her tactics had been successful and she proudly informed her spouse that she was now writing 'to tell you I am not breeding (is not that clever)'.[20] Others, according to Rueff, exchanged information with their women friends.

> But the issue of their termes returning, when they know they
> are free and delivered from the Feature, they impart and
> communicate likewise those murthering arts and cruell
> practices to others, that thereby many murthers of sillie
> Infants are committed.[21]

Such desires for control of their bodies were castigated by Dryden in his rendition of Juvenal's *Satyrs* (1693):

> You seldom hear of the Rich Mantle, spread
> For the Babe, born in the great Lady's Bed:
> Such is the Pow'r of Herbs; such Arts they use
> To make them Barren, or their fruit to lose.
> But thou, whatever Slops she will have brought,
> Be thankful, and supply the deadly Draught:
> Help her to make Manslaughter; let her bleed,
> And never want for Savin at her need.[22]

The value of such passages, in which men sought to denigrate the woman's desire to control her fertility as a manifestation of evil, is clearly limited. Nevertheless they unintentionally give some sense of the courage of the woman intent on limiting births.

A second reason to induce miscarriage was in order to avoid the misery brought on by too large a family. Dr Buchan was of the opinion that the lower orders, if they were to be called upon to reproduce, had to receive some charitable support from the community. He was quoted by Tytler:

'This would make the poor esteem fertility a blessing, whereas many of them think it is the greatest curse that can befall them.' To this Dr. Underwood adds, that 'he has known them express thankfulness when their children are dead.' The reason of which in some measure may be, that it is frequently mentioned as a matter of reproach to a man in low circumstances, that he has a large family. And in this country, it is usual with such persons to consult apothecaries, quacks, and old women, for medicines to make their wives barren.[23]

Children could, if they reached a working age and found employment, be an incalculable asset for the working-class couple. But if their birth jeopardized the health of the mother their arrival could be viewed with fear. As physician to the Manchester Infirmary John Ferriar spoke from first-hand experience when he described the trials faced by some of the poor:

A young couple live very happily, till the woman is confined to her first lying-in. The cessation of her employment then produces a deficiency in their income, at a time when expenses unavoidably increase. She therefore wants many comforts, and even the indulgences necessary to her situation: she becomes sickly, droops, and at last is laid up by a fever, or pneumonic complaint; the child dwindles, and frequently dies. The husband, unable to hire a nurse, gives up most of his time to attendance on his wife and child; his wages are reduced to a trifle; vexation and want render him at last diseased, and the whole family sometimes perishes.[24]

In such a context it should have occasioned little surprise if some working-class families sought protection from an unwanted birth by recourse to abortion.

A third reason for the married to have recourse to abortion was in order to end the childbearing career of the woman once she neared menopause. A number of historians have noted that the spacing of births of married English women lengthened from their mid-thirties on. This could be attributed to either declining fecundity or reliance upon some form of birth control.

In *The Family Life of Ralph Josselin: A Seventeenth Century Clergyman* Alan Macfarlane speculates that the series of miscarriages experienced by Josselin's wife once they already had five living children was not merely coincidental.[25] In his diary entry of 8 December 1661 Josselin wrote 'my wife very apprehensive shee breeds again', on 22 December, 'my wife if breeding feareth miscarrying', and on 23 December 'at night my wife miscarried, of a false conception, a mercy to bee free of it, and I trust god will preserve my deare ones life'.[26] Whether or not Josselin's account suggested that the conception was unwanted and the miscarriage induced is not entirely clear but the passages are suggestive. Jane Josselin's series of miscarriages occurred when she was forty and presumably losing her enthusiasm for childbearing. Each occurred, moreover, as soon as she discovered that she was pregnant. A similar scenario can be followed in the remarkably candid letters of Edward and Henrietta Stanley.[27] Henrietta Stanley married at a relatively early age and by thirty-six had given birth to nine children. Three child-free years then passed but on 5 November 1847 she warned her husband, then in London, by letter 'I have put Demoniacal affairs in another note.' In what terms she described her unwanted pregnancy and her views on terminating it we can only guess from the response made by her husband:

> My Dearest Love – This Last misfortune is indeed grievous & puts all others in the shade. What can you have been doing to account for so juvenile a proceeding, it comes very opportunely to disturb all your family arrangements & revives the nursery & Williams in full vigour. I only hope it is not the beginning of another flock for what to do with them I am sure I know not. I am afraid however it is too late to mend & you must make the best of it tho' bad is best.

It is especially interesting to note how Edward Stanley attributed to his wife the entire responsibility for determining family size. Clearly Henrietta Stanley assumed she had the right to take appropriate measures. On 9 November she wrote: 'Dearest Love – A hot bath, a tremendous walk & a great dose have succeeded but it is a warning.' Her husband replied: 'I hope you are not going to do yourself any harm in your violent proceedings, for though it would be a great bore it is not worth while playing tricks to escape its consequences. If however you

are none the worse the great result is all the better.' Henrietta
Stanley's last words to her husband on the subject were 'I was
sure you would feel the same horror I did at an increase of
family but I am reassured for the future by the efficacy of
means.' How many other couples had similar conversations
about recourse to abortion we can only guess.[28] It seems likely,
however, that when such discussions did take place the same
sorts of topics would have to have been touched on: the burden
placed on the health of the mother and the economy of the
household by an additional birth; the possible dangers of
attempting to induce a miscarriage; and the responsibility of
the woman to take the final decision.

Who would assist women seeking abortions? Some have
already been mentioned in passing. The man responsible for
the seduction of the unmarried woman frequently sought out
for her the necessary herbal abortifacient. With married
women the help of female friends and spouses was called upon.
What captivated the attention of observers, however, was the
figure of the abortionist. Here again the evidence must be
treated with some caution. The vast majority of abortions were
no doubt self-induced or aided by a woman friend but the
diabolical figure of the professional abortionist hypnotized
commentators. In past generations midwife abortionists were
closely associated with witchcraft. In 1438 John Nider attacked
the 'wicked practices' of midwives in provoking miscarriages.[29]
The authors of the *Malleus Maleficarum* (1488) asserted 'That
witches who are Midwives in Various Ways kill the Child
Conceived in the Womb, and Procure an Abortion; or if they do
not do this Offer New-Born Children to Devils'.[30] In 1566
Elizabeth Frauncis was accused of witchcraft for giving blood to
Satan in return for a drug to procure abortion, and in 1637 Rueff
warned women, 'that they use not Wicked Arts and policies of
old Witches and Harlots, for removing and punishing of
whom, the care and charge ought most specially to belong to
Magistrates, to wit, being the Fathers of the People'.[31] The last
in the line of these abortionist witches was Mary Bateman, the
'Yorkshire Witch'. Although she was executed for murder in
1809 her original notoriety was based on her ability to use
sympathetic magic to 'screw down' the enemies of her clients
and her expertise as an abortionist.[32]

By the late seventeenth century accusations of witchcraft
were diminishing and abortionists were now mainly accused

of acting simply out of a desire for monetary gain. In 1664 Pepys accused Dr Alexander Fraser of being an abortionist by attributing his wealth and power at court to the aid he provided courtesans 'in helping to slip their calfes when there is occasion'.[33] In *The Compleat Midwife's Practice Enlarged* (1698) John Pechey warned his readership that those associated with delivering mothers had to avoid carefully any action that might make them liable to being charged with abortion. Pechey backed up his argument by citing the words of the famous French midwife Louise Bourgeois:

> Above all things, you must beware (for any treasure in the world) of adhering to one vice, such as they are guilty of who give Remedies to cause Abortion; for those that do ill, and those that seek a damnable remedy, are wicked in a high degree. But it is a higher degree of wickedness for those that are no way ingaged in the business, for lucres sake to kill both the body and the soul of an infant. This I do not speak that thou shouldest refuse to give Remedies upon just occasions: but to take heed how you be cheated by subtle persons, who shall tell you fine stories of the diseases of their Wives, or Daughters, which they may say are very honest, hoping to get from you some Receipts to effect their wicked designs.[34]

By the eighteenth century Defoe was referring in *Moll Flanders* to abortionists with vast clienteles; in *Augusta Triumphans* he spoke of women depending upon 'a set of Old-Bedlams, or pretended Midwives, who make it their trade to bring them off for three or four Guineas'.[35] Grose reprinted an advertisement placed by one such practitioner in the *Morning Post* of 18 April 1780: 'Any Lady whose situation may require a temporary retirement, may be accommodated agreeable to her wishes in the house of a gentleman of eminence in the profession, where honour and secrecy may be depended on, and where every vestige of pregnancy is obliterated'.[36] William Buchan's suspicions were such that he wrote, in *Domestic Medicine or the Family Physician*, 'I have never heard without shuddering any advertisement of temporary retreats, or pretended accommodations for pregnant ladies.'[37]

Apothecaries were portrayed by many as being likely providers of abortifacients. One of the versions of 'Mary Hamilton' portrayed the seducer as a pottinger or apothecary. Quaife reports a seventeenth-century case: 'A married man tried to persuade the aunt of a girl he had seduced "to buy something at the apothecaries and give it to her kinswoman to destroy her conception." When the aunt refused he pleaded directly with the girl "to take something to take away her child within her".'[38] Samuel Garth presented in his poem *The Dispensary* (1699) the druggist whom

> Poor pregnant Lais his advice would have,
> To lose by art what fruitful Nature gave.[39]

And to turn from the world of fiction to that of fact one finds in the mid-eighteenth century the Duchess of Devonshire saying of the recent miscarriage of Lady Clermont, 'to tell you the truth, as it is pretty certain Mr Morden the apothecary was the father, I fear some wicked method was made use of to procure abortion, and that is more likely as Mr Morden might bring the drug from his own shop'.[40] Abortionists were thus not unknown in early modern England but they would be turned to only by those who could afford their services and only after the woman's attempts to induce her own miscarriage had failed.

By what means would women procure an abortion? There are four main types found in early modern England: by magic, by physical means, by pessary and by herbal potion. The magical would include attempts at employing sympathetic magic to reverse a conception. So in Spenser's *The Faerie Queene*, for example, the old nurse is portrayed as muttering prayers, and

> That sayed, her round about she from her turnd,
> She turned her contrarie to the Sunne,
> Thrise she her turnd contrary, and returned,
> All contrary, for she the right did shunne,
> And ever what she did, was streight undonne.
> So thought she to undoe her daughters love.[41]

Some in Cambridgeshire believed up until the late nineteenth century that touching a dead man's finger or keeping corpse money – a florin placed on a dead body until burial – could prevent the births of children. Sowbread (*Panis porcinus*) was reported in the sixteenth and seventeenth centuries 'for the natural attractive virtue' it enjoyed to provoke abortion in women walking over it. In more than one herbal one can find the ditty:

If over it a child-great woman stride
Instant abortion often doth betide.[42]

The same amulets that protected a woman from miscarriage could, if worn in the appropriate place, also cause a miscarriage. Accordingly, Sowerby stated that if jasper stone or eagle stone were tied to the thigh early in gestation they could – like sowbread – draw down the embryo.[43]

In the category of physical means of provoking abortion came bleedings and beatings. In one seventeenth-century case a young woman was asked by her lover 'to bruise her body thereby to destroy the . . . child'.[44] More common were reports of a seducer beating a woman in order to cause her miscarriage. Bleedings of the thighs and feet which some doctors thought could assist in labour were turned to by others in attempts at premature expulsion.[45] One also finds reports of women indulging in various forms of strenuous exercises from dancing to carrying heavy burdens for the purposes of terminating a pregnancy. Tight lacing, which was to be reproved by many moralists, had as one of its purposes the provoking of abortion. Thus Rueff condemned those that, 'make the first experiments by lacing them in themselves strait and hard, that they may extinguish and destroy the feature conceived in their wombe'.[46]

The third type of abortive method – the use of a pessary – linked physical and herbal means. In a 1450 edition of what has been called the first English gynaecological handbook there is a recipe for such a pessary.

> Also the root of iris put into the womb or fumigated underneath makes a woman lose her child, for iris roots are hot and dry and have the virtue of opening, heating, consuming, and wasting. For when a woman is feeble and the child cannot come out, then it is better that the child be killed than the mother of the child also die.[47]

In the sixteenth- and seventeenth-century herbals a variety of such pessaries were described. *Acorus* or *Gladen*, mixed with vinegar and placed in the matrix, was said never to fail; 'Floure de luce, the roote with honey put in as a pessary, doeth cause abortion' reported a second author; and Stinking Gladden, asserted a third, 'profiteth being used as a pessarie, to provoketh the terms, and will cause abortion'.[48] The most

extensive list was provided by Leonard Sowerby who suggested packing the womb with unwashed wool, or the roots of
sowbread, gentian, ploughman's spicknard and madder.[49]
Exactly how these pessaries were supposed to work is not
always clear. In India and South America midwives can precipitate a miscarriage by carefully inserting a twig of the erukka
or parsley plant into the cervix.[50] Presumably the English
manuals were suggesting similar stratagems but the humoral
idea of heating the womb and the magical idea of drawing
down the embryo were also present.

The fourth and most popular method employed by past
generations to cause abortion was a herbal potion. Women, in
pursuit of abortifacients, had recourse to almost every type of
toxic and non-toxic substance. Indeed, Taussig noted in his
classic *Abortion, Spontaneous and Induced* that much early
medical knowledge about toxicology was drawn from women
experimenting on themselves with various drugs and potions.
The fact that between the seventeenth and nineteenth centuries
the slang term for pregnant was 'poisoned' reflected in part the
association of toxic substances with attempts to end unwanted
pregnancies.[51]

But was every woman whose periods had stopped and who
employed a herbal potion seeking to abort? Or were some
simply seeking cures for amenorrhoea? The fact that many
recipes were described as useful to 'restore the menses' could
be taken to mean that their consumers were not seeking abortions. It should be noted, however, that women in past times
would seldom use the term 'abortion' except when describing
an inducement of miscarriage *after* 'quickening', an issue
discussed below. A researcher in contemporary Jamaica has
reported that there too twentieth-century island women

> rarely confronted the idea of pregnancy termination but
> tended to speak of 'bringing down the period' when it had
> not 'been seen' for a while. Similarly, the prescription for
> using marigold boiled with cerasee directed, 'If menstru-
> ation ceases, drink as tea for nine mornings'.[52]

In seventeenth- and eighteenth-century women's receipts
books a similar reluctance to discuss abortion *per se* is found.
Instead one finds extensive suggestions on how to 'provoke the
terms', 'purge the courses', 'bring down the flowers' and deal
with 'menses obstructed'. In the early 1600s Ann Brumwich

recommended ale and horehound 'to bring them [the menses] down when they stope in young maides'; in 1647 Lady Sleigh prescribed herbgrace in wine; Lady Miller preferred aloes and syrup of mugwort; Johanna St John, aloes and gentian; Miss Frances Springatt, saffron in wine. In the early eighteenth century Letitia Owen described the efficacy of a pennyroyal purge, Abigail Smith in 1725 prescribed 'for to procure the monthly termes of a woman' orange in white wine and Mrs Finger boasted of her own recipe that 'it hardly ever fails but has brought the same person about two or three times'.[53]

In almost every published medical herbal one can also find lists of potions to induce menstruation. In *The Regiment of Life* (1544) Jehan Goeuriot described how savin and hellebore 'provoke the menses' as did Andrew Boorde in *The Breviary of Helthe* (1547).[54] William Langham in *The Garden of Health* (1578) listed 'Peniroyall', rue and savin as able 'to bring down the flowers' and Sir Kenelm Digby recommended in *Choice and Experimental Receipts in Physicke and Chirgery* (1675) sulphur of antimony 'to bring down a Woman's Course'.[55] In the eighteenth century Elizabeth Smith gave recipes in *The Compleat Housewife* (1725) for 'An Opening Drink' of penny-royal and another 'To procure the Menses' of pennyroyal and myrrh.[56] At the end of the 1700s John Gregory spoke in his *Medical Lectures* (1770) of savin to restore the menses, Henry Manning proposed an emmenagogue of aloes in *A Treatise on Female Diseases* (1775) and even John Wesley included in *Primitive Physicke* (1776) treatment for 'Menses Obstructed' with pennyroyal and Black Hellebore.[57] The same ingredients for the same purposes were listed in A. Hume, *Every Woman Her Own Physician or, the Lady's Medical Assistant* (1776) and John Aikin, *A Manual of Materia Medica* (1785).[58] During both the seventeenth and eighteenth centuries savin and penny-royal appear to have been the two most frequently prescribed herbs and at the end of the period they are ranked as the most powerful 'provokers of the catamenia' in the anonymous *Complete Herbal or Family Physician* (1787) and in the 1798 edition of *Nicholas Culpeper's English Physician and Complete Herbal*.[59] Clearly, many of these potions were used simply to 'restore the menses' but it is equally obvious that some women also employed them for the purposes of inducing miscarriage. On occasion even those authors who provided information on such concoctions sought to dissuade their readers from turning their new-found knowledge to self-serving purposes. James Primerose in *Popular Errours* (1651) castigated those who sought by bleedings or 'physick' to expel a foetus and John Sadler in the *Sick Woman's Private Looking Glass* (1636) cautioned 'Ignorance makes women become murderers to the fruit of their owne bodies'.[60]

Although almost all the writers of herbals explicitly condemned herbal abortifacients, many described, in addition to menstrual potions, recipes which could be used to provoke miscarriages. The herbs to which they attributed abortifacient powers included: aloes, angelica, alexander, absinthe, bistort (snakeweed), chervil, clary, calamint, cannabis (hemp), calomel, dittany, eringo, ergot of rye, ground pine, hellebore, mugwort, mustard, mithridate, madder, marigold, oak leaves, pennyroyal, parsley, rue, southernwood, savin, saxifrage, thyme and tansy. The three most famous herbal abortifacients were ergot of rye, pennyroyal and savin. In England the serious medical investigations of ergot of rye or 'spurred rye' (*Claviceps purpurea*) took place in the first decades of the nineteenth century. Christison mentioned that its use to induce miscarriages or precipitate births was known to quacks and midwives in Germany from at least the seventeenth century and in France from the eighteenth. An 'oxytocic' agent that helps contract the smooth muscles of the uterus, ergot of rye is mentioned in some of the early herbals but its use in England seemed to spread only in the late eighteenth and early nineteenth centuries.[61] It was eventually to be taken over by doctors and in the alkaloid form of ergometrine is still employed by obstetricians as a uterine stimulant.

Pennyroyal (*Mentha pulegium*), a member of the mint family, is mentioned by the herbalists more frequently than ergot of rye, both to induce menstruation and as an abortifacient. Thus in a seventeenth-century text this emmenagogue was described as being able to expel 'ye Embrya' and in an eighteenth-century work, to 'provoketh womens courses'.[62] In twentieth-century Norfolk large doses have continued to be recommended to procure abortion.[63]

Savin (*Juniperus sabina*) enjoyed the reputation of being the most powerful of abortifacients. This small bush related to the juniper took its name from the Sabines, the ancient Italian race, but so associated was it with abortion that the 1886 *Dictionary of Plantnames* stated that its appellation derived from its 'being able to save a young woman from shame': hence it was known in Galloway as a 'Saving-Tree'.[64] It was employed by the Romans but in the early modern period was first mentioned in the *Malleus Maleficarum* of 1488: 'without the help of devils, a man can by natural means, such as herbs, savin for example, or other emmenagogues, procure that a woman cannot generate or conceive'.[65] In 1572 Margaret Manister of Essex was accused of incest with a brother-in-law. After her affair she 'drank saven, and that night fell sick and so was the whole week after'.[66] In a similar case reported in 1574 the rector of Leaden Roding in Essex went to London to buy savin for his seduced maid.[67] In a 1578 herbal it was said able to 'driveth down the termes'; a 1657 text claimed that it 'causeth Abortion in those that take it before they have gone their full time, and therefore, as I have said, it is not permitted to those whom you suspect to desire it for any such occasion, as some Harlots doe'.[68] In an early eighteenth-century discussion it was described as 'under Mars, and kills worms, provokes the Terms, and destroys the fruit of the Womb'; in a 1787 work as 'a powerful provoker of the catamenia, causing abortion, and expelling the birth'; and in a 1790 study as 'if given to women with child, causes abortion'.[69]

Savin's notoriety was such that it won a place in the literary world. In *The Faerie Queene* Spenser portrayed the seduced woman turning to the aged nurse who

> Had gathered Rew, Savine, and the flowre
> Of Camphora, and Calamint, and Dill,
> All which she in a earthen Pot did poure,
> And to the brim With Colt wood did fill,
> And many drops of milke and bloude through it did spill.[70]

Abraham Cowley spoke in 1640 of 'fatal Sabina nymph of infamy', Dryden referred in 1693 to the woman who should 'never want for savix for her need,' and Thomas Middleton in *A Game at Chess* (1624) presented a character lamenting the fact that,

> And when I look,
> To gather fruit, find nothing but the savin-tree
> Too frequent in nun's orchards, and there planted
> By all conjectures, to destroy fruit rather.[71]

There are indeed several references to savin bushes being

planted and cared for by women for the explicit purpose of providing the necessary leaves. A nineteenth-century doctor reported that villagers still considered savin valuable.

> Popular opinion is decidedly in its favour, and it is the medicine most commonly employed to procure criminal abortion. Dr Davis, in his elaborate work, mentions on the testimony of one of his pupils, who served his apprenticeship at Tonbridge, that in the neighbourhood of that town there was a remarkably fine savin tree the decoction of the leaves of which was successfully used, not only to remove menstrual suspension, but also to induce abortion.[72]

The numerous references to abortifacient herbs provides evidence that they were not only widely available, but frequently employed.

Help in inducing a miscarriage was not only found in herbals and recipe books. The eighteenth century witnessed the beginnings of the commercialization of abortion, as of contraception. 'Female pills' appeared on the market for the purposes of 'restoring the menses' just as condoms began to be sold for protection from venereal disease and prevention of conception.[73] The oldest pill was Dr Patrick Anderson's Scot's Pill, consisting of a compound of aloes and jalop, which appeared in 1635 and was still sold in the twentieth century. The most popular were John Hooper's Female Pills which were patented in 1743. Hooper, an apothecary and male midwife from Reading, advertised his pill as a cure for hysteria and stomach disorders. They were probably composed of ferrous sulphate, aloes and myrrh. Iron enjoyed a reputation as an abortifacient and Hooper's 'female pills', containing iron, were the first in a long line to be employed for the purpose of inducing miscarriage. Later competitors included Widow Welch's Pills, Fuller's Female Benedictine Pills, Mr Sherratt's Female Pills and the Restorative Salo Pills of Mrs Milner who also offered lying-in services.[74] The majority of women could not afford such products and would continue to rely on their own gardens or local herbalists for their needs. The appearance of these new pharmaceuticals implies, however, that by the latter half of the eighteenth century there was emerging a middle-class, urbanized type of woman who, cut off from the traditional world of female medical lore, would have to rely increasingly on apothecaries and doctors for medication.[75]

Did these abortifacients work? Some obviously did either by directly affecting the uterus or by indirectly bringing on a miscarriage by poisoning the mother.[76] Edward Shorter has provided the fullest account of the issue and concludes that the effectiveness of many of the potions will never be fully determined.[77] We do not know all the drugs employed, nor in what forms or quantities. We have not yet investigated the specific abortifacient actions of the complete pharmacopoeia employed in early centuries. And finally we are not sure if some women who thought they had found a successful abortifacient were in fact pregnant or, if they were, miscarried for reasons unrelated to the use of the medicine. For our purposes, however, the vast range of references to herbal abortifacients is chiefly of interest because of the light it casts, not on the rate of successful induction of abortions, but on the reality of a widespread tradition of women seeking to limit births by herbal means.[78]

The final and most important question to ask about abortion in early modern England is how was it viewed by the women who had recourse to it? It is a difficult question to answer. In some cultures abortion has been explicitly condoned. In ancient Greece, for example, it was argued that the practice was legitimate if the couple were over-age or the child incestuously conceived.[79] In some parts of Africa the fact that a woman was still nursing one child was sufficient reason to terminate an additional pregnancy.[80] In England the view of women seemed to be that the legitimacy of the act of abortion was related to the context in which it took place. If abortion allowed a pre- or extra-marital relationship to go undetected it could be considered an evil inasmuch as it was tainted by the more general issue of promiscuity. This explains why married women were so often the witnesses against the unmarried who had recourse to either abortion or infanticide. But when abortion was employed by the married woman for the purposes of protecting the health and well-being of herself and her family the practice could have, in the eyes of the female community, some basis of justification. It was, however, more than a question of who aborted and why they aborted; it was also a question of *when* they aborted. Right up until the twentieth century many women assumed that abortion was neither a crime nor immoral as long as it was self-induced and took place before 'quickening'. A careful analysis of the concept of 'quickening' is thus necessary if attitudes towards abortion in the seventeenth and eighteenth centuries are to be fully understood.

During this period the traditional view was sustained that the foetus went through various stages of development. According to Aristotelians the foetus was 'animated', at about the fourth month, to Christians 'ensouled', and to most laymen 'quickened'. What had been potential now became actual life. So we find in the Anglo-Saxon leechbooks or medical texts the statement: 'In the third month he [the foetus] is a man without a soul. In the fourth month he is firm in his limbs. In the fifth month he is quick and waxeth'.[81] Wyclif's English translation of the Bible (I Kings XVII, 22) ran: 'The soul of the child is turned agen with ynn hym, and he agen quickened'.[82] Jehan Palsgrave wrote of a woman that 'She quickynned on al hallon day'.[83] In *The Arte of Rhetorique* Thomas Wilson referred to 'Hym that killeth the child so sone as it beginneth to quicken'.[84] Christopher Hooke in *The Child-birth or Woman's Lecture* (1590) declared that it was a great loss for women not to bear children: 'that is either being conceived, they shall not be quickened: or being quickened, they shall not in the womb accomplish the just time of the birth'.[85] In *A Discourse on Civil Life* (1606) Lord Bryskett followed Aristotle in describing the embryo before animation as being little more than a vegetable: 'it is the creature unperfect in the wombe, whiles it is betweene the forme of seed, and of the kind whence it cometh'.[86] Stephen Blancard in his *Physical Dictionary* followed the same line of thought in explaining that the embryo was 'the Rudiment of a Child in the Womb' and only called a foetus when made perfect.[87] It was for this reason that James Guillemeau argued that a miscarriage in the first forty days could not be called an abortion, but simply a 'shift or a slipping away'.[88] John Maubray agreed that the foetus was formed and organized around the fiftieth day, but declared that animation only occurred between the seventieth and the hundredth.[89] Aristotle and his popularizers like Venette asserted that the two sexes developed at differing speeds with the males being ensouled at forty-five days and the females at fifty; the former moving at three months and the latter at four.[90] Thomas Denman, one of the leading experts in eighteenth-century midwifery, placed quickening at around fifteen weeks.[91] So did the midwife who informed William Byrd of Maryland that twenty weeks would pass 'from the time a woman is quick when she will seldom fail to be brought to bed'.[92]

The importance of quickening drew the attention of poets. In *Othello* Shakespeare spoke of 'summer's flies . . . That quicken even with blowing'; referring similarly to the animal world, John Ray mentioned spawn that 'would be lost in those seas, the bottom being too cold for it to quicken there'; and Richard Blackmore declared in *Prince Arthur* that:

Barren Night did pregnant grow,
And quicken'd with the World in Embrio.

In coarser language Thomas Urquhart translated Rabelais's use of the term *vitault* (meaning penis) as 'quickening-peg'.[93]

Until the late eighteenth century both lay people and doctors employed the term quickening, but not always for the same purposes. For medical men it simply signified the woman's consciousness of the stirring of the new being in her womb and was merely the final indication of her pregnancy. For women quickening meant that the embryo now had life and its destruction would be a sin. By the same token some women would use the belief that *prior* to quickening life was not present in order to legitimate their inducement of early miscarriage. Women's belief that they had the right to do whatever necessary to bring on a period prior to quickening appears to have had a long history in the western world. Procopius informs us that the Empress Theodora, finding herself pregnant,

did everything to accomplish, in her usual way, an abortion, but she was unsuccessful, by all the means employed, in killing the untimely infant, for by now it lacked but little of its human shape. Consequently, since she met with no success, she gave up trying and was compelled to bear the child.[94]

In short, after quickening attempts at abortion ceased. For the woman who faced an undesired pregnancy it would signify her defeat. Thus Samuel Pepys wrote in his diary for January 1663 of the King's mistress, Lady Castelmain, who 'quickened at my Lord Gerard's dinner, and cried out that she was undone; and all the lords and men were fain to quit the room, and women called to help her'.[95]

Given the fact that only the woman herself knew if she had quickened the concept gave a good deal of discretion to the individual of deciding whether or not she should have recourse to herbal purgatives.[96] But in the eighteenth century this view came increasingly under attack from medical men and moralists. The eighteenth-century Italian doctor of theology Cangiamila asserted that though Gregory XIV reserved excommunication only for those who aborted *after* quickening, it was nevertheless the duty of priests to teach 'that it is never permitted to procure abortion, even before the foetus is animated. . . . Nothing is more unreal than the false and dangerous subtlety that distinguishes the animated foetus from the one that has not received life'.[97] Women, asserted Cangiamila, clung to the notion of a lack of vitality before quickening because it allowed them to proceed with the abortion free of remorse. In France Dr Des-Essartz claimed that by the 1760s priests, philosophers and scientists were all agreed that the foetus was alive from the moment of conception. The task was now to instruct women: 'Could not we reasonably hope that mothers will abjure the error that holds that the child only has life towards the third or fourth month?'[98] In eighteenth-century England doctors expressed the same concerns. Women who sought abortions in the first months of gestation assumed it was their right. A dramatic portrayal of such a claim was contained in Daniel Defoe's *Conjugal Lewdness*. He presented a woman making the assertion

> that all the while the *Foetus* is forming, and the Embrio or Conception is proceeding, even to the Moment that the Soul is infused, so long it is absolutely not in her Power only, but in her right, to kill or keep alive, save or destroy the Thing she goes with, she won't call it Child; and that therefore till then she resolves to use all manner of Art, to the help of Drugs and Physicians, whether Astringents, Diureticks, Emeticks, or of whatever kind, nay even to Purgations, Potions, Poisons, or any thing that Apothecaries or Druggists can supply: But she goes farther. . . . If Drugs and Medicine fail her she will call to the Devil for help, and if Spells, Filtres, Charms, Witchcraft, or all the Powers of Hell would bring it about for her, she would not scruple to make use of them for her resolved Purpose.[99]

Though eighteenth-century doctors and moralists talked about the vitality of life from the moment of conception, women clung to the traditional view that life was not present until the foetus quickened. They could thus choose to regard themselves not as pregnant, but as 'irregular'. This brings one back to the discussion of women's recipes for inducing menstruation. While doctors increasingly condemned abortifacient measures women themselves would say that they were taking such potions, not to abort, but to bring on a period. Such actions would be more 'thinkable' for the eighteenth-century woman than for her nineteenth-century counterpart: a wide variety of herbal remedies were at hand; doctors' ability to detect the existence of foetal life was hardly superior to that of their patients; and the inducement of miscarriage was not made a statutory crime until 1803.

The history of abortion in early modern England has received little attention possibly because it has been assumed that its danger to a mother's health and its immorality would have made the practice unthinkable to all but the most desperate. This chapter has sought to show, first, that concerns for health and family well-being could have led many to contemplate abortion; second that there existed a wide range of techniques that were believed to be effective in precipitating miscarriages; and third that the concept of 'quickening' permitted women to consider the action as legitimate. For these reasons we have to conclude that abortion played a far more important role in the regulation of fertility in past generations than has usually been believed.[100] The extraordinary number of references in herbals and recipe books to potions designed to 'restore the menses' provides further evidence that women were not passive in relation to their fertility; they wanted to control it and were willing to go to considerable lengths to do so.

In the pattern of reproductive rituals that we have been attempting to uncover abortion figures centrally; a study of the practice reveals the existence and the tenacity of a separate female sexual culture. But women's desires to control their own fertility did not go unchallenged. In the sixteenth century Andrew Boorde, in describing the cause of abortion, cautioned: 'it may become by recipes of medicines as by extreme purgations, potions, and other laxative drinks, of the which I dare not to speak of at this time lest any light woman should have knowledge by the which willful abortions should happen'.[101] Two centuries later Henry Bracken expressed the same sentiments:

> I shall not enter into an Account of the Methods, or rather Tricks, practised by some vile women, in order to bring on *Miscarriages*, for fear of being guilty of telling such something

that would do it; yet they sometimes meet with their Desert; for by their dangerous Experiments, they frequently lose their Lives.[102]

The ultimate victory of such opponents of abortion came with the criminalization of the practice, the subject of the following chapter.

5
'Converting this measure of security into a crime':
the early nineteenth-century abortion laws

Missionaries campaigned vigorously against a number of measures by which women controlled their fertility, including the segregation of the sexes after childbirth, the whole practice of polygamy, and women's secret societies used for, among other things, initiation in traditional methods of fertility control.
Barbara Rogers, *The Domestication of Women: Discrimination in Developing Societies* (1980)

Anthropologists tell us that the intrusion into traditional cultures of western doctors' elaboration of scientific explanations of the process of procreation can, in the short term, lead to lay persons becoming 'ignorant' of the functioning of their own bodies. It was suggested in chapter one that such a process could be detected in eighteenth-century England as a new biomedical explanation of procreation diverged from older Galenic beliefs. The result was the splitting of a once common sexual culture. This chapter tests the argument that a similar process took place as new sanctions – justified by medical discoveries – were levied against abortion at the beginning of the nineteenth century. Our hypothesis is not simply that in making abortion a statutory crime the ruling classes were asserting their rights to police the reproductive actions of the lower orders but also that the real significance of the legislation lay in the fact that it revealed special interest groups undermining traditional reproductive rituals as they pursued self-serving ambitions.

One view of birth control in the nineteenth century is that it consisted simply of the passing down by the upper classes of contraceptive knowledge to the lower classes. This glosses over the fact that a variety of traditional forms of fertility control were already available to the masses and that the century opened with Parliament criminalizing perhaps the most important – abortion. In 1803 abortion became a statutory crime for the first time in English history; in 1828 and in 1837 the law was revised and strengthened. The passage of such statutes set a legal precedent but it would be wrong to suggest that this was the first time that public opinion sought to control the fertility of individual women. As has been shown in previous chapters, husbands and wives always had to take into account at some conscious or unconscious level the wishes of the outside community when planning their family strategies. But clearly there was a qualitative difference between a society in which fertility decisions were affected by traditional informal sanctions and one in which such decisions could be deemed criminal acts.[1]

Why were these laws not passed until the beginning of the nineteenth century? It has been argued that they did not appear earlier because only in the 1800s did large numbers of women have recourse to inducement of miscarriage. It is possible that an increase in their numbers might have drawn the attention of the authorities to a practice which they then sought to police. Unfortunately there is no quantitative way of substantiating such an argument. One does not know how many nineteenth-century women sought to end their pregnancies. There is also the problem of explaining why it was that though observers in the seventeenth and eighteenth centuries made repeated references to employment of abortifacients by both the single and the married, their reports did not result in the passing of earlier repressive legislation. Without denying the possibility that there was an increasing incidence of recourse to abortion at the beginning of the nineteenth century, it seems safest to conclude that the early nineteenth-century anti-abortion laws are primarily of interest in what they tell us about changes not in fertility control behaviour, but in the attitudes towards such behaviour of those who had a hand in the law-making process.

It is clearly too simplistic a notion to believe that because prior to 1803 abortion was not a statutory offence it was considered, in the eyes of the ruling orders, an unexceptional occurrence but suddenly at the turn of the century was viewed by them with horror. To place the passage of the abortion laws in context this chapter will first sketch out the background to the eighteenth-century religious, legal and medical arguments concerning inducement of miscarriage. It will be shown that though clerics, jurists and medical men condemned abortion they also condoned the practice to some extent. In other words, abortions were declared evil in principle but the lack of effective sanctions against the practice implied a degree of toleration.

In the second part of this chapter, two processes will be shown to have led in the late eighteenth and early nineteenth centuries in an unanticipated fashion to legal sanctions against abortion. The first was the campaign by humanitarians and jurists to reform the law against infanticide which by its very success in having infanticide treated more leniently was balanced by having abortion treated more severely. And the second was the campaign launched by doctors as part of the process of their professionalization to eliminate both rival practitioners such as midwives and their nonscientific concepts such as quickening.

Abortion was first and foremost a moral issue. The history of the Catholic Church's views on abortion have received exhaustive analysis from scholars such as John Noonan but little has been written about the issue in England either before or after the Reformation.[2] Although the apocryphal works did refer to the practice, there was no reference in either the Old or the New Testaments to volitional abortion. Given such lacunae national traditions were obviously important. English clerics who referred back to the early Church fathers found the practice repeatedly condemned because of the Christian fear of the fate that awaited the unbaptized infant. This doctrine was promulgated by Origen whose temper can be judged from the fact that he followed literally the suggestion that the blessed were those who 'made themselves eunuchs for the kingdom of heaven's sake'.[3] In his *Origines Ecclesiasticae* Joseph Bingham cited a number of other early Church fathers similarly hostile to inducement of miscarriage. In the Canons of St Basil it was declared: 'Let her that procures abortion, undergo ten years' penance, whether the embryo be perfectly formed or not'. Tertullian thundered:

In the prohibition of murder we are forbidden to destroy the conception in the womb, whilst the blood is in its first formation of a human body. To hinder that which might be born, is but an anticipation or hastening of murder: and it is all one, whether a man destroy that life which is already born, or disturb that which is preparing to be born. He is a man who is in a disposition to be a man; and all fruit is now in its seed or principle of existence.[4]

St Jerome similarly referred to women 'drinking of barrenness, and murdering of infants before they were born'.[5] In combining infanticide, abortion and contraception as equal forms of murder these early ascetics set a rhetorical line that would be followed by some canonists, but was obviously difficult to impose on the secular world.[6] That such teachings were carried to England is evident from a reading of Robert of Brunne's *Handlyng Synne* (1303).

> If men or women be so wild
> To frustrate the getting of a child
> Once it is begotten, with word or deed
> With Meat or drink that they do eat,
> Or other means that it die,
> Than they do a very great folly;
> With slaughter thou has hidden thereby
> So that your lechery is not known;
> In evil thou art greatly culpable
> In two sins, and damnable.[7]

Similarly, in *The Canterbury Tales* Chaucer had the parson explain:

> Eek if a womman by necligence overlyeth hire child in her slepyng, it is homycide and deedly synne./ Eek whan man destourbeth concepcioun of a child, and maketh a womman outher bareyne by drynkknge venenouse herbes thurgh which she may nat conceyve, or sleeth a child by drynkes wilfully, or elles putteth certein material thynges in hire secret places slee the child,/ or elles dooth unkyndely synne, by which man or womman shedeth hire nature in manere or in place there as a child may nat be conceived, or elles a woman have conceyved, and hurt hirsef and sleeth the child, yet it is homycide.[8]

Even the teachings of the humanist Erasmus were cited by

Thomas Wilson in *The Arte of Rhetorique* (1553) to provide proof of the evil of abortion:

> There is no nation so savage, nor yet so hard harted, within the whole world, but the same abhoreth murderying of infantes and newe borne babes. Kynges also and hedde rulers, dooe likewise punishe most streightly, all suche as seke meanes to be delivered before their tyme, or use Phisicke to ware barren, and never to beare children. What is the reason? Marie thei compt small difference betwixt hym, that killeth the child, so soon as it beginneth to quicken; and thother, that seketh all meanes possible, never to have any child at all.[9]

Wilson's work was followed thirty-five years later by perhaps the most famous condemnation of abortion, the papal bull *Effraenatum* (20 October 1588) of Pope Sixtus V.

> Who does not abhor the lustful cruelty or cruel lust of impioys men, a lust which goes so far they procure poisons to extinguish and destroy the conceived foetus within the womb, even attempting by a wicked crime to destroy their own offspring before he lives, or if it lives to kill it before it is born? Who, then, would not condemn with the most severe punishments the crimes of those who by poisons, potions, and *maleficia* induce sterility in women, or impede by cursed medicines their conceiving or bearing.[10]

These various condemnations of abortion might appear to be comprehensive, but in fact they contained a number of loop-holes. In the first place the Church canons retained the concept of 'ensoulment' that held that vitality was present in the male only after forty days and in the female after eighty. As later commentators were to complain, this permitted women to claim that life was not present before quickening in defending their use of potions. In the second place the condemnations were not as strict as they might at first appear because their target was often not so much the act of abortion *per se* as much as the illicit relationship that led up to it or the reliance on magical herbs or *maleficia* that were employed to procure it.[11] Indeed as far as Catholics were concerned no outright condemnation of abortion was produced by canonists until the nineteenth century. The Cult of the Immaculate Conception – made an obligatory celebration by Pope Clement XI in 1701 –

was important, as John Noonan has pointed out, in directing the eighteenth-century Church towards a more absolutist line. If Mary was immaculate when conceived presumably she, and therefore everyone else, necessarily would have to be alive from the moment of conception. Accordingly the casuistry of Sanchez and Liguori had to be dropped by canonists along with the forty/eighty day concepts of ensoulment. Only in 1854, when Pius IX declared Mary free of sins from the point of conception, was the final foundation for the Church's complete condemnation of abortion at any stage of gestation secured.[12]

But what view did English Protestants take of abortion, freed as they were from following the Catholics' devotion to Mary? Puritan pronouncements appear to have differed little from those of Catholics. Gouge declared that, compared to those who used contraceptives,

> they who purposely take things to make away with their children in their wombe, are in a farre higher degree guilty of bloud: yea even of wilfull murther. For that which hath received a soule formed in it by God, if it bee unjustly cast away, shall be revenged.[13]

In *An Exposition of the Moral Law* (1636) John Weemse dealt with the practice in a section entitled 'On murther in general'. He reminded his readers of the Biblical penalties levied against a man whose actions cause a miscarriage:

> 'How pretious a thing is the life of man in the sight of God.' *Exod.*, XXI, 22.
> If *they follow no mischief*, that is, if the child be not figured, yet, as the Greeke hath it, or not a living soul as yet, yet the striker was mulcted or amorced, and this was paid to the husband; not onely for the wrong done to the woman, but also for the wrong done to that which should have become a child, although he was not as yet *foetus signatus*. . . . It is a great cruelty to kill the child in the mothers belly, to kill this innocent in his first mansion, which should have beene the place of his refuge, the tunicle in which he is wrapped in his mothers belly, is called *shilo*, because (as the Hebrews say) the young infant should live peaceably in it, in his mothers wombe, as a place of refuge.[14]

The Protestant attack on abortion – like the Catholic – was not as clear-cut as it first appears. Life was not thought by Protestants to be present at the moment of conception. According to Weemse the seed 'curdled' on the seventh day, the foetus was perfected on the forty-fifth, stirred on the ninetieth and the baby born in the ninth month.[15] For both Weemse and Gouge abortion only occurred after ensoulment, and Weemse only considered cases in which a woman miscarried as a result of a beating from a man.

The ambiguous position occupied by abortion in the catalogue of sins was further demonstrated by the ways in which religious sanctions were levied against it. In the medieval handbooks of penance the penalties charged against those who aborted varied according to the stage in gestation. In an Irish penitential of 800 it was declared that

> A woman who causes miscarriage of that which she has conceived after it has become established in the womb, three years and a half of penance. If the flesh is formed, it is seven years. If the soul has entered it, fourteen years' penance.

According to the Penitential (668–9) of Theodore of Canterbury,

> Women who commit abortion before [the foetus] has life, shall do penance for one year . . . and if later, that is, more than forty days after conception, they shall do penance as murderesses, that is, for three years.[16]

The penalties sound severe (especially those for the unmarried which were to be three times those for the married), but it is doubtful whether they were acted upon. Moreover, to put these charges in context it should be noted that simple 'fornicators' were supposed to do penance for seven years which implies that early abortion was viewed as having only half the moral obliquity of an illicit relationship.

By the sixteenth century the ecclesiastical courts or 'bawdy courts' were responsible for dealing with such matrimonial and sexual problems. Their judgements were not without importance, but the courts were restricted to dealing with moral offences and could only impose 'penances' – usually a fine and public confession.[17] In the court records there are many references to incontinence, prostitution, bastardy, incest and venereal disease, but very few to abortion. Some references were found in sixteenth-century Hampshire court records to persons committing abortions and providing herbal remedies.[18] Paul Hair reported a few other cases in *Before the Bawdy Court*:

London, 1527. Margaret Sawnders is charged that with potions she killed an infant in the womb of Joan Byrde. She appears and his lordship orders her and Joan Byrde to be sworn and to reply truthfully to the charge, and Joan Byrde denied it.

Harpenden, Hertfordshire, 1530. Item, 'we charge you John [Hunt] that you have advised this woman Joan [Willys] and persuaded her to obtain and *certayn drynkes to destroy the childe that she is with.'* His lordship warned him to appear, and he admitted that he had known her carnally, at which his lordship ordered that on a Sunday to be fixed he should perform a public penance before Harpenden Cross in the normal way . . .

Stokenchurch, Buckinghamshire, 1530. Joan [Schower] tells the midwives that she has been carnally known by William [Hewes] and impregnated but took a medicine to bring about an abortion. And she has two children before for which lesser crime she was punished.

Durham, 1535. Elizabeth Johnson against Agnes Cutter, *for defamation*, viz. that this plaintiff should give her daughter suche drinkes as did slee the childe that she was with.[19]

What is interesting in almost all the cases cited is that abortion by itself was rarely the cause of the prosecution. It was not the woman who aborted, but rather the promiscuous woman, or the seducer, or the provider of abortifacients who was tracked down. In short it was public scandal associated with abortion that forced the courts into action; the woman privately seeking to induce her own miscarriage would not be the source of such a commotion and would correspondingly be rarely cited.[20]

From the early seventeenth century on even fewer cases of abortion were reported as compared to the sixteenth century. This was due in part to the fact that Protestants were opposed to casuistry and accordingly reluctant to prolong the detailed analysis of types of moral misdemeanours so beloved by Catholic canonists. Moreover the ecclesiastical courts themselves were closed by the Roundheads between 1641 and 1660. The courts were revived during the Restoration, but by then had lost most of their vigour.[21] Their demise signalled the triumph of the common law courts whose advocates asserted that the church courts threatened property rights by meddling in family matters such as those touching on tithes and testaments.[22]

Donald Veall has likened the triumph of the common law courts in matters relating to property as a manifestation of the splitting of sin and crime, two vices which the ecclesiastical courts had confused. Indeed, in the late 1640s it could be said that in England there was no such thing as a sexual crime. The authorities soon decided, however, that to avoid public disorder morality had in some instances to be buttressed by legal sanctions.[23] Accordingly in 1650 incest and adultery were made crimes.[24] In this context it is interesting to note that another 150 years would pass before abortion was made a statutory crime. It was not totally ignored, however, and to understand its legal position in the intervening period it is necessary to turn to the writings of the common law advocates.

In Bracton's *Pleas of the Crown* (1250) the judicial view of the practice of abortion followed closely that of the religious. 'If one strikes a pregnant woman or gives her poison in order to procure an abortion, if the foetus is already formed or quickened, especially if it is quickened, he commits homicide'.[25] The woman who precipitated her own miscarriage was clearly not taken into account but rather only the man who after quickening caused such an action. Fleta's late thirteenth-century gloss on Bracton did implicate the woman:

> He, too, in strictness is a homicide who has pressed upon a pregnant woman or has given her poison or has struck her in order to procure an abortion or to prevent conception, if the foetus was already formed and quickened, and similarly he who has given or accepted poison with the intention of preventing procreation of conception. A woman also commits homicide if, by potion or the like, she destroys a quickened child in her womb.[26]

By the seventeenth century, however, the notion of such deeds being similar to murder was dropped. Edward Coke in *The Third Part of the Institutes of the Laws of England* (1644) declared: 'If a woman be quick with child, and by a Potion or otherwise killeth it in her wombe; or if a man beat her, whereby the child dieth in her body, and she is delivered of a dead childe, this is a great misprison and no murder.'[27] A similar line was taken by Matthew Hale in *Pleas of the Crown* (1682):

> It [the child] must be a person in *rerum natura*. If a Woman quick with Child take a potion to kill it, and accordingly it is destroyed without being born alive [it is] a great misprision,

121

> but no Felony; but if born alive, and after dies of that potion, it is Murder.[28]

Seventeenth-century jurists thus recognized that a woman could be charged with procuring her own abortion, but only after the foetus had quickened. Its seriousness in the eyes of the law is difficult to judge. A 'misprision' was a non-capital common law offence and included a number of treasonous acts such as bribing a witness, attacking a judge or drawing blood in the king's presence.[29] Abortion after quickening was possibly included in this category because an aborting woman might have been perceived as treasonably depriving either her husband or the community of a child.

The eighteenth-century legalists continued the seventeenth-century stress on quickening but when categorizing abortion increasingly replaced the term misprision with the more explicitly lenient term misdemeanour. Blackstone, in his *Commentaries on the Laws of England* (1765), asserted,

> Life . . . begins in the contemplation of law as soon as an infant is able to stir in the mother's womb. For if a woman is quick with child, and by a potion or otherwise, killeth it in her womb; or if any one beat her, whereby the child dieth in her body, and she is delivered of a dead child; this, though not murder, was by the antient law homicide or man-slaughter (Bracton). But Sir Edward Coke doth not look upon this offence in quite so atrocious a light, but merely as a heinous misdemenor.[30]

Similarly *The Laws Respecting Women* (1777) noted: 'As soon as an infant is able to stir in its mother's womb, it becomes an object of protection in the eye of the law; therefore if a woman is quick with child, and by a potion or otherwise she killeth it in her womb . . . [it is] a great misprision only'.[31]

What did this mean in practice? Abortion was considered a common law misdemeanour only if it were procured after the stage of quickening, that is about four months after conception. As the woman herself was the only one to know if she had quickened and as attempts at abortion after four months would be rare, the law was in effect a dead letter. A search of the *Select Trials* of the Old Bailey turns up a large number of eighteenth-century cases of other 'moral crimes' such as rape, sodomy, infanticide and bigamy but none of abortion.[32] The fact that abortion originally lay within the jurisdiction of the by then nearly moribund ecclesiastical courts could explain in part the indifference of the common law courts to the issue. But for whatever reason neither set of courts made any great effort to prosecute abortion in the eighteenth century.[33] Lawyers and churchmen were theoretically opposed, in any event, only to abortions occurring after quickening and they refrained from seeking to penalize earlier actions which might affect what in their eyes could only be considered *potential* life. Doctors, who composed the one other professional group which one might anticipate being preoccupied by the subject, had their own specific concerns to consider regarding this issue and these must now be analysed.

In seventeenth- and early eighteenth-century medical texts one finds the practice of abortion condemned in much the same language as that found in the works of moralists. It was only in the latter half of the eighteenth century that the medical discussion of inducement of miscarriage began to differ markedly from that of the religious or the judicial. But if a new medical perspective on the vitality of foetal life began to emerge this did not lend to a simplification of the issue. To appreciate fully medical men's discussion of the termination of pregnancies it has to be recalled that such issues involved their professional as well as their moral preoccupations. The resulting tension was perhaps best demonstrated by the defence of therapeutic abortion made by some of the very doctors who were most hostile to non-therapeutic or, in their words, 'criminal' abortions. This double-edged concern surfaced as part of the eighteenth-century upsurge of medical interest in obstetrical and gynaecological problems.

A good deal has already been written about doctors' entry into what previously had been deemed a woman's realm – midwifery.[34] The emergence of male midwives and the creation of lying-in hospitals were the most obvious demonstrations of this new concern of doctors with the problems associated with pregnancy. The most dramatic example of surgeons' assertion of competence in this new field was provided by their discussion of how to proceed in those cases where safe delivery was impossible and only the life of the mother or child could be assured. Such a quandary was posed when, for example, rickets and osteomalacia distorted a woman's pelvic passage to such an extent that a natural birth was impossible. Particularly plagued were 'females in a low situation', wrote one doctor, 'who have had children in quick succession'.[35] Bearing and nursing children could diminish the under-nourished mother's calcium and phosphorus reserves so softening and distorting the bones of the pelvic region. It was a cruel irony that such a fate was met by many poor women who had purposely extended their nursing as long as possible in the very hopes of avoiding a further conception. We know today that lactation does produce post-partum amenorrhoea but even in the seventeenth and eighteenth centuries it was common knowledge that '. . . long suckling of children', in William Petty's words, was a 'hindrance to the speedier propagation of mankind'.[36] Unfortunately not all who nursed were so protected from a subsequent conception. Some women would thus find themselves debilitated by nursing while pregnant. If often repeated the practice could prove dangerous. 'A female', warned Dr John Hull, 'who gives suck during her pregnancy and is at the same time indisposed or ill fed, which is not uncommon amongst the lower classes, must suffer in a still greater degree from the expenditure of ossific material'.[37] It was the opinion of Denman, the leading late eighteenth-century obstetrician, and others that the problem was compounded by the emergence of factory labour.

> Formerly the cases in which the Caesarean operation could come to be considered were almost universally confined to cities, or very large towns, where the customs and manners of life most frequently occasioned, with every other kind of decrepitude, distortions of the pelvis and all its consequences. But within these few years, from the general dissemination of manufacturers, especially that of cotton, over many parts of the country, these evils have become much more frequent; and as the children employed in them are obliged to stand, or are confined to one posture for many hours together, before their bones have acquired sufficient stability to support them, many have become deformed. To boys it may be a great evil and a mortification to have bandy legs, yet this does not prevent their becoming fathers; but the girls under the same circumstances must often be precluded from being mothers; nor could they go through the process of parturition without infinite suffering and danger.[38]

It is difficult to determine the accuracy of such statements – the fact that more doctors were in the towns would mean that the medical complications of urban women were more likely to be discovered than those of the rural – but it is true that a disproportionate number of nineteenth-century Caesarians carried out as a consequence of pelvic deformities took place in the textile regions of Lancashire.[39]

To prevent such complications doctors advised poor working women that to protect themselves they should avoid frequent conceptions (they did not say how), shorten nursings and improve their diets, in particular by taking ling-liver oil. Impoverished women would obviously be in no position to act on such counsels. What could be done when a deformed woman reached the latter stages of pregnancy? Should one have recourse to the Caesarian operation which, given ignorance of infection, meant almost certain death for the mother, or should one sacrifice the child in hopes of saving the woman? The first Englishwoman to survive a Caesarian was Jane Foster of Lancashire operated on in 1793 by Dr James Barlow.[40] The most vocal defender of the operation was Dr John Hull, like Barlow a pupil of Charles White, founder of the Manchester Lying-In Charity. Hull appears to have been somewhat of a showman eager to make a name for himself. 'He had been practising midwifery since the age of seventeen and had delivered quintuplets in 1786, all stillborn, which he pickled and presented to John Hunter'.[41] Hull's attempts at the Caesarian operation in 1794 and 1798 were equally unsuccessful and led to a violent attack on the procedure as cruel and unnecessary by William Simmons of the Manchester Infirmary. Simmons had the English medical tradition on his side inasmuch as the majority of surgeons felt that the Caesarian was only justifiable if the death of the woman had already occurred or was unavoidable; in any other case recourse had to be made to therapeutic abortion. The importance of the Hull–Simmons controversy which predated the 1803 abortion law by a few years was that it provided a useful summing-up of eighteenth-century English attitudes towards the 'rights' of the mother, the foetus and the doctor.[42]

Although there were reports of successful Caesarians from the Continent – especially France – from the sixteenth century on, a long line of English medical men starting with William Harvey, Percivall Willughby and Sir Richard Manningham refused to consider the sacrifice of the mother for the child as morally defensible. If the pelvic passage of the woman was too narrow to promise a safe delivery other strategies were preferred. The first was induction of miscarriage or premature labour by rupture of the membranes.[43] John Burns, a lecturer in midwifery at Glasgow, stated that 'tapping is, sometimes, with great propriety, done at a particular period, in order to avoid a greater evil. It is now general opinion, that contraction will unavoidably follow the evacuation of the waters'.[44] The induction of premature labour by rupture of the membranes was a key English (and Scottish) contribution to obstetrics and indeed was long referred to as 'the English method'. It was suggested and employed by Macauley in 1756 and popularized by Thomas Denman and Samuel Merriman. Although it could in some cases result in the safe delivery of an undersized baby, the fact that the operation was based on the calculated decision of risking the child for the sake of the mother led to its being opposed by the French on religious grounds. Only after 1830 was it practised in Paris. The second and more radical form of therapeutic abortion used by the English in the last stages of pregnancy was craniotomy. A crochet was employed to end the pregnancy and remove the foetus.[45]

In this context the importance of English doctors' discussion of the relative merits of therapeutic abortion is that in it they spelled out what they saw as their legitimate right to terminate a pregnancy. In so doing they declared as their first interest the health of the woman. In the repeated attacks made on the Caesarian by men such as Ould, Osborn and Denman it was made clear that the rights of the woman always took priority over those of the foetus.[46] Correspondingly, in order to justify therapeutic abortion, doctors went to great lengths to deny the foetus the possession of real life. William Osborn, physician to the London General Lying-In Charity Hospital, asserted that even at the last stages of pregnancy the child could experience neither pleasure nor pain, and that the mother herself could only begin to love the child in any meaningful way sometime after its birth. A miscarriage would be regretted by the wealthy family as involving the loss of a 'representative' but in general the death of an unborn child was not to be severely regretted:

To society, likewise, the loss of any individual child, must be exceedingly small, when it is known by daily observation, what great numbers of children are stillborn, or die without such violence before death; when it is likewise known, how very precarious is the chance of a child's living two years; but how most of all precarious, is its arrival at that period of life, when it can be of any service to his fellow-creatures, or even participate itself in the enjoyments of the world.[47]

William Hunter concurred: 'The life of the mother . . . is almost of an incomparably greater value than that of an unborn child; a being which we may suppose has no enjoyment, and has neither a desire to live, nor fear to die'.[48] It was, declared Simmons, 'a pretty commonly received opinion, that the life of the child, before birth, resembles the state of vegetable life; and, that the disproportionate bulk of its nervous system to the other parts of its body is not intended to increase its sensibility, but to answer important purposes after birth'.[49]

Did religion have any role to play in determining the value of embryonic life? In France in 1733 a theological conclave at the Sorbonne laid down guidelines justifying recourse to the Caesarian.[50] In England, however, doctors from 1756 on agreed amongst themselves and without the benefit of religious counsel on the legitimacy of therapeutic abortion. Physicians from Ould in 1742 to Merriman in 1822 attributed the continental penchant for the Caesarian to Catholic preoccupations with the sanctity of foetal life.[51] In contrast English doctors claimed that they were motivated solely by medical concerns and the laws of nature. Nature always sacrificed the embryo for the mother and accordingly Denman asserted that inducement of miscarriages was 'no more than an imitation in one case of what happens spontaneously in another'. It was the doctor's duty to avoid futile religious arguments and get on with the business in hand. 'True religion and the common sense of mankind appear to have nothing contradictory. The doctrine they teach of its being our duty to do all the good in our power, and to avoid all the mischief we can, is applicable to the exigencies of every state, and we may be easily reconciled to it on the present occasion'.[52]

It should be noted, however, that though English doctors would consider therapeutic abortion because of medical reasons they would not tolerate the idea of their patients resorting to such practices. Denman, one of the most vocal defenders of therapeutic abortion, was also one of the first to warn against the immorality of its repetition. He argued that if

127

a woman could not safely deliver the law should permit the dissolution of her marriage to prevent 'the moral turpitude of conceiving children without the chance of bringing them living into the world'.[53] When a woman had already been provided with two or three abortions and had conceived once more, Denman suggested that though the Caesarian section meant almost certain death, she should be subjected to the operation. In the mid-nineteenth century Radford argued that a woman should be permitted only one abortion before facing the ordeals of the Caesarian.[54] In America a crippled Irishwoman, Mrs Reynolds, having had two births aborted, was warned by her surgeon, C. D. Meigs, that her next would be by Caesarian. She was so operated on in 1835 and survived, conceived, and was operated on again successfully in 1837. This remarkable woman, whose obstetrical career can be followed in the nineteenth-century American medical journals, did not die until 1885, having, one is pleased to note, outlived all the medical notables of Philadelphia who exposed her to such terrors in the 1830s.[55]

What can one conclude from this late eighteenth-century debate over the relative merits of Caesarian section and therapeutic abortion? It is clear that doctors considered therapeutic abortion in certain cases a justified practice – and that they alone should judge the physical dangers posed the woman and decide on its necessity. If it were deemed necessary no outsider, not even a husband, could interfere since, Denman asserted, such interference would be 'contrary to the rights and interests of society, and never could have satisfied the mind, or justified the conduct of any person who should have submitted to be governed by it'.[56] But the second point to stress is that though doctors defended a specific operation, it was deemed justifiable only if doctors carried it out. Abortions provided by irregular practitioners for non-medical reasons were increasingly castigated at the end of the eighteenth century. Farr lamented in 1788 the fact that infanticides were punished while abortion, 'this crime, which is practised generally by the most abandoned escapes punishment'.[57] Denman ended his 1794 discussion of induction of premature labour with the warning: 'But concluding all the observations which it seems necessary to make on this subject, I solemnly deprecate their being applied to dishonest and immoral purposes'.[58] Similarly Merriman lamented: 'It ought not to be concealed, that it [abortion] has been had recourse to by wicked and unprincipled persons, for the atrocious and criminal purpose of procuring abortion: and sometimes has been unnecessarily adopted by the ignorant or incautious'.[59]

Given the facts that the ecclesiastical courts, which in the first instance dealt with abortion cases, were by the eighteenth century nearly moribund, that the common law courts were also refusing to try such cases and that English doctors were even advancing arguments in favour of therapeutic abortion, it is difficult at first to provide an explanation for the passage of the acts that made abortion a statutory crime in 1803 and tightened the law in 1828 and 1837. The mystery is deepened when one finds that the precedent-setting 1803 bill elicited no debate. It was introduced into Parliament by Lord Ellenborough, a firm believer in the use of the law as terror. His Maiming and Wounding Bill was submitted after only five days' notice and in all created ten new capital offences. It placed the crime of abortion for the first time on a statutory basis.[60] In section one the statute generally followed tradition in holding that the use of poisons with the intent to procure the miscarriage of a woman 'quick with child' was a felony. In treating as a felony a practice previously considered a misdemeanour, a marked shift occurred but the real innovation of the statute was in section two in which it was held that *before* quickening abortion by poison or 'any instrument' was also a crime. In other words the attempt to provoke a miscarriage in the first four months after conception was now for the first time in English history declared to be a criminal act.

Why did the abortion laws appear when they did? To answer this question one's first impulse is to look for a preceding discussion of abortion in the last decades of the eighteenth century. One does not find such a directly related debate but rather two processes that indirectly set the stage for the passage of such legislation; first, the campaign by humanitarians for the reform of the law on infanticide, and second, the effort launched by doctors, as part of the process of their professionalization, to eliminate both rival practitioners such as midwives and their non-scientific concepts such as quickening.

Infanticide, like abortion, was dealt with in the Middle Ages by the ecclesiastical courts though on occasion an infant murder might be sent on to the criminal assizes. Prior to the sixteenth century few cases of infanticide were either reported or looked for.[61] Under the Tudors, however, the upper orders' growing preoccupation with the social threat posed by the poor led to a new concern for their moral lives.[62] The fear that poor, promiscuous women were foisting their illegitimate offspring onto the parish led to the inclusion in the 1576 Poor Law of a section which required single mothers to declare publicly the names of the fathers of their children. The intent of the law was to shift the burden of the care of the illegitimate child from the parish back to the purported father but in practice its first consequence was to disgrace the mother by publicizing her immorality. To avoid the humiliation and social ostracism that might result many women accordingly concealed their pregnancies. Some even went so far as to commit infanticide; the assumption that all single women who concealed their conceptions might harbour such plans led to additional legislation in 1624.[63] The act 'to prevent the murdering of Bastard Children' began with the preamble

> Whereas, many lewd women that have been delivered of bastard children, to avoid their shame, and to escape punishment, do secretly bury or conceal the death of their children, and after, if the child be found dead, the said women do alledge, that the said child was born dead; whereas it falleth out sometimes (although hardly it is to be proved) that the said child or children were murthered by the said women, their lewd mothers, or by their assent or procurement:
>
> II. For the preventing therefore of this great mischief, be it enacted by the authority of this present parliament, That if any woman after one month next ensuing the end of this session of parliament be delivered of any issue of her body, male or female, which being born alive, should by the laws of this realm be a bastard, and that she endeavour privately, either by drowning or secret burying thereof, or any other way, either by herself or the procuring of others, so to conceal the death thereof, as that it may not come to light, whether it were born alive or not, but be concealed: in every such case the said mother so offending shall suffer death as in case of murther, except such mother can make proof by one witness at the least, that the child (whose death was by her so intended to be concealed) was born dead.[64]

This extraordinary statute created not a new crime, but a new way to deal with an old crime. Infanticide was made a unique charge in English law inasmuch as a single mother who concealed her pregnancy and whose child subsequently died now had to prove her innocence of murder; the court did not have to establish her guilt.[65] It should be stressed that only some mothers – the unmarried or 'lewd' – were subject to the law, the presumption being that the married would not be forced to such extremes. It would have been impossible, of course, to have extended such surveillance to the married but such an omission suggested that the statute was more a response to a fear of promiscuity than a reaction to a threat to infant life.

The infanticide law was from the first objectionable and unworkable. Judges and juries were naturally reluctant to sentence to death poor, single women for crimes that were only circumstantially proven. And even in cases where the burden of guilt was overwhelming the courts would rarely convict because of the public hostility to such a process in which women suffered while their seducers escaped.[66] Juries simply refused to convict and seized upon any evidence to bring down an innocent verdict. If there were no signs of violence, if the woman were poor, if some accident to the child might have happened, if some scrap of baby's clothing in the woman's possession suggested she intended on keeping the child after its concealed birth, her chances of acquittal were good.[67] Juries in effect ignored the statute and accepted the fact that infanticide, if it occurred, was the result of exceptional circumstances, frequently complicated by the mental instability of the mother.

The statute remained on the books, however, and for almost 200 years evoked increasingly heated debate. There were some who defended the statute. The anonymous author of *A Rebuke to the Sin of Uncleanness* (1704) was pleased to note that promiscuity brought 'an intollerable Shame with it, as we see in the Case of those Women who have barbarously murdered their own Off-Spring to cover the Shame of their Defilement'. In William Walsh's 'A Dialogue Concerning Women' a character called Misogynes wanted the law to go even further, 'Go but one circuit with the Judges here in *England*; observe how many Women are condemned for killing their Bastard children'.[68] But few writers openly declared themselves in support of such a barbaric law and the chorus of voices hostile to the statute

131

increased over time. Robert Burton in *The Anatomy of Melancholy* (1621) anticipated Montesquieu by drawing on cross-cultural evidence to show how in some societies infant-icide was accepted as an understandable response to the problems posed by poverty.

> In *Iaponia* 'tis a common thing to stifle their children if they bee poore, or to make an abort, which *Aristotle* commends. In that civill commonwealth of *China*, the mother strangles her childe, if shee bee not able to bring it up, and had rather loose, then sell it, or have it endure such misery as poore men doe.[69]

That ordinary seventeenth-century English women appre-ciated the lengths to which unwed mothers could be pushed by poverty was demonstrated by a riot in 1658. A woman had been hanged for infanticide but when taken to be anatomized was revived by the doctors. The bailiffs seized her and hanged her again. 'The Women', a contemporary report read, 'were exceedingly enraged at it, cut downe the tree whereon shee was hanged'.[70]

In the eighteenth century the attack on the infanticide statute was based on two main arguments; first that the law was unfair and unworkable, and second that the medical evidence employed in such cases was unreliable. The most famous portrayal of the law in action occurred in Sir Walter Scott's *The Heart of Mid-Lothian* (1818) in which Effie Dean's illegitimate baby disappears and she is faced with being convicted as a murderer. Scott built up his plot on a foundation laid by eighteenth-century law reformers. Bernard de Mandeville asserted that the law of infanticide, even if it could prevent mothers from killing their new-born children, would only lead them to escape their fates by other stratagems, 'either by destroying the Infants before their Birth, or suffering them afterwards to die by wilful Neglect'.[71] Blackstone, usually so detached, declared that the statute 'savors pretty strongly of severity'.[72] In 1772 Edmund Burke and Charles James Fox, the most impressive speakers in the Commons, combined to call for the repeal of 21 James I, c. 27.

> They said that in the case of women having bastard children, the common [and] statute laws were inconsistent; that the common law subjected to a fine, to a month's imprisonment,

and the flagellation; that this institution necessarily rendered the having of a bastard child infamous; that the statute law, in opposition to all this, made concealment capital; that every mother, who had not at least one witness to prove, that her child, if it was dead, was born dead, or died naturally, must be hanged; that nothing could be more unjust, or inconsistent with the principles of all law, than first to force a woman through modesty to concealment, and then to hang her for that concealment; . . . that nothing could more strongly prove the absurdity and inexpediency of the law, than the impossibility of putting it in execution, under which the judges found themselves; that the laws were made to be executed, not dispensed with.[73]

The same line of reasoning that held that such laws not only unjustly deprived the individual of the right of self-defence, but because of their lack of enforcement led to the public's contempt for all laws, was followed on the continent by Montesquieu and Beccaria.[74] Brissot noted that in infanticide cases as in abortion it was only the poor who were ever detected. The more atrocious the laws levied against them the less likely were such laws to be successful.

The best advice that one can give to a legislator on the subject of this crime [abortion], is to attempt to prevent rather than to punish it. The danger that an abortion always poses a mother, independent of this love for her children which nature always inspires, will make this a rare crime, provided that the Civil Laws wisely seek to abet her natural penchants.[75]

Jeremy Bentham was of the same opinion that individual calculations of possible pleasures or pains inevitably determined whether infanticide or abortion would be carried out. The law in meddling in such areas could only make matters worse.

The laws against this offence [infanticide], under pretence of humanity, are a most manifest violation of it. Compare the offence with the punishment. The offence is what is improperly called the death of an infant, who has ceased to be, before knowing what existence is, – a result of a nature not to give the slightest inquietude to the most timid imagination; and which can cause no regrets but to the very person who, through a sentiment of shame and pity, has refused to prolong a life begun under the auspices of misery. And what is the punishment? – the barbarous infliction of an ignominious death upon an unhappy mother, whose very offence proves her excessive sensibility; upon a woman guided by despair, who, in hardening her heart against the softest instinct of nature, has harmed no one but herself![76]

Reformers who attacked the infanticide statute because of its general violations of common justice were supported by some medical men who attacked the specific ways in which the act led to the employment of medical evidence. If a child were born dead the mother clearly should not be convicted of its murder. Accordingly, determining whether or not it had breathed was essential in many cases. A traditional way of establishing this was for a doctor to determine whether the lungs of the dead child would float. If they did it was presumed that the child had been born alive and its subsequent death therefore had to be explained by the mother. In the latter half of the eighteenth century the validity of such findings was questioned. The *Gentleman's Magazine* carried a letter in 1774 from 'W.P.' who asserted that a learned gentleman had refuted the claim of Dr Gibson that such tests were infallible.[77] Any suspicions regarding the nature of these tests, the anonymous writer claimed, had to lead to great caution because the lives of 'many poor unhappy women' depended on such judgements.

A fuller critique of the lung test was provided in 1784 in the posthumously published tract of William Hunter entitled *On the Uncertainty of the Signs of Murder in the Case of Bastard Children*. William Hunter, as the most famous eighteenth-century British investigator of the processes of gestation and parturition, clearly spoke from long experience. He provided an eloquent defence of unmarried mothers which combined both medical knowledge and compassion. It was his belief that few infanticides were ever cases of simple murder. Many seduced women would rather destroy themselves than their child and were only prevented by the fear of the shame they would bring to their families. A concealment of an illegitimate birth was a natural and understandable ploy but it was always possible that a woman bearing in secret would swoon and awake to find her child dead. The custom of assuming that concealment of the birth was proof of the intent to commit premeditated infanticide was, according to Hunter, in most cases unfounded. But turning to his true area of competence – medical surgery – Hunter concluded his argument by attacking the process of determining viability by the testing of lungs. He showed that it was possible for the lungs of a child which had been born dead to float. It followed that the test was simply not reliable and should not be introduced in such important cases. When the question was whether or not a woman would be put to death, Hunter argued, her innocence had to be assumed unless there was overwhelming evidence to the contrary.[78]

It was in this context that the infanticide law was finally reformed in Lord Ellenborough's omnibus Maiming and Wounding Bill of 1803 (43 Geo. III, c. 58). Ellenborough was moved to act, however, not out of any great concern for unmarried mothers, but because of his fear that the continual flouting of the statute was undermining respect for the law. He therefore suggested relaxing the law on infanticide,

> to relieve the judges from the difficulties they labour under in respect to the trial of women indicted for child-murder, in the case of bastards. At present the judges were obliged to strain the law for the sake of lenity, and to admit the lightest suggestion that the child was stillborn as evidence of the fact.[79]

Under the new act the woman who concealed the birth of an illegitimate child, even should it be found dead, would no longer be assumed to be guilty of infanticide. She could, however, if the circumstances surrounding the death were suspicious, be tried for murder. But the proof of her guilt would now have to be established, as in any other murder case, by the prosecution. The old burden of the woman proving her innocence was removed though she still might be tried for concealment of birth and subject to a maximum punishment of two years in a house of correction. Given the great difficulty of proving child murder it was the latter sort of charge which would be increasingly laid.[80] Ellenborough was obviously motivated not by compassion, but by the desire to penalize women, if only with minor penalties, rather than have the courts appear to condone their actions by refusing to convict.

For the purpose of this study what is of chief importance is that Ellenborough's 1803 bill on the one hand repealed the infanticide law, but on the other made it a felony punishable by

death to administer poison 'to cause and procure the miscarriage of any woman then quick with child', and a felony
punishable by fine, imprisonment, pillory, whipping or trans-
portation to attempt by drug or instrument to procure the
miscarriage of any woman 'not being or not being proved to be
quick with child'.[81] Why these sections on abortion were added
to the 1803 statute is not clear, especially when the practice was
lumped in with other crimes such as firing a gun and administering poison with intent to kill and burning down one's house
with intent to defraud insurers. It would appear that
Ellenborough, as a confirmed conservative, was determined to
make the law on abortion more stringent to balance the fact that
in the same statute the law on infanticide was made less harsh.
He repealed a capital crime in one section and created another
in the next. Bentham was of the opinion that it was ironic that
judges who recognized the futility of employing the death
penalty in infanticide cases should now turn it to the purposes
of policing abortion.

> Of any of the known measures that can be employed to
> procure abortion danger, more or less considerable to health
> is a consequence, and lest this danger should not be great
> enough, legislators, with their usual barbarity, have stepped
> in and converted this measure of security into a crime.[82]

But what Bentham overlooked was that though the infanticide
law was aimed at mothers, the abortion law was aimed not
directly at mothers but at those who might assist them in
procuring abortions. Indeed a reading of the statute suggests
that the abortion sections were directed more at the crime of the
murder of women by the purveyors of purported abortifacients
than at the act of abortion *per se*. Such an interpretation was
borne out by the fact that the Maiming and Wounding Bill dealt
with a variety of forms of murder and attempted murder.[83] The
implication was that abortion was just another form of murder
in which the victim was not the foetus but the woman. Burnett
asserted in 1824 that it had been the rising number of deaths of
women brought on by the use of poisonous abortifacients
which led to the passage of the bill in 1803. 'This practice
became so general, and the effects of it so fatal, that of late years,
the arm of the law has been exerted strongly against it.'[84]
According to Sir Edmund Head the villain was the seducer: 'it
is the man who generally suggests the crime which, while it

aims at prematurely destroying the child, puts the life of the mother herself in peril'.[85] The argument that the statute sought as much to protect women as to end abortion was further substantiated by the fact that if a woman sought to induce her own miscarriage no law was broken. A contributor to the *Legal Examiner* concluded in 1832: 'a careful examination has not convinced us that the law, either common or statute, makes a voluntary abortion a felony or misdemeanor, nor any other operation, although accompanied with risks of self-destruction'.[86]

Women who sought to procure their own abortions were thus not to be directly subjected to the sanctions of the new law. But how would doctors fare, especially those who defended the necessity of therapeutic abortion? Given the fact that the inducement of miscarriage was the *only* operation which by statute was a felony, such doctors were vitally implicated. They were especially preoccupied by the fear that lawyers were presuming to speak on issues in which doctors had to be concerned. Indeed, the abortion law discussion after 1803 was in a sense a test of the professional standing of medicine. It was in part due to the pressure of doctors, or so some of them claimed, that the abortion law was revised in 1828 and 1837.

From the number of medical critiques that attacked the 1803 law it was clear that the statute was drafted without consultations being made by the Lord Chancellor with the medical fraternity. Doctors were unhappy with the act of 1803, but what sort of statute did they seek? They desired first and foremost that non-medical personnel who provided abortions be tracked down. In 1815 Bartley attacked those who actually employed public advertisements to lure women patients to their dens.[87] In his 1816 edition of *Domestic Medicine* Buchan declared: 'Those wretches who daily advertise their assistance to women in this business deserve, in my opinion, the most severe of all human punishments.'[88] Hutchinson in 1820 declared that abortionists represented 'an evil of the highest magnitude; for they are often persons with whom it is familiar, and who make the commission of it a sort of regular profession'.[89] But while doctors sought the repression of those irregular practitioners who provided abortions they fretted that the law did not specifically exempt from prosecution surgeons carrying out similar acts. Burns in 1806 defended 'those necessary attempts which are occasionally made to procure premature labour, or even abortion, where the safety of the mother demands this interference'.[90] The fact that the law referred to those who 'unlawfully' procured abortion was hopefully cited by some doctors as evidence that the statute implicitly recognized the legitimacy of the act in some situations. The *Lancet* similarly suggested that the law made no mention of the use of instruments after quickening for the reason of sparing *accoucheurs* who might otherwise be prosecuted.[91] Others such as Ryan, however, bewailed the vagueness and confusion of the law and wanted explicit provisions made for therapeutic abortions.[92]

As far as the women who sought abortions were concerned doctors seemed to be content that they continued to be treated at best as mere accomplices. The risks they ran in seeking to induce miscarriage were sufficient punishment. One finds in Buchan's 1816 edition the passage:

> Every woman who procures an abortion does it at the hazard of her life; yet there are not a few who run this risk merely to prevent the trouble of bearing and bringing up children. It is surely a most unnatural crime, and cannot even in the abandoned, be viewed without horror; but in the decent matron, it is still more unpardonable.[93]

Smith noted, as had Buchan, that abortion was sought by those seeking to avoid illegitimate births and 'also from an unnatural desire to avoid the inconvenience of childbearing, and even for the purpose of preserving personal symmetry'.[94] Smith was one of the few to demand that women be charged as accomplices. Most doctors tended to trivialize the woman's role and attribute her actions to ignorance. Radford typically bemoaned the ignorance of women that prevented them from appreciating the fact that even before quickening they carried 'a living human being', a *'potential man'*.[95]

The main problem with the 1803 law on abortion as far as doctors were concerned was not that it did not explicitly discuss therapeutic abortion, nor that it spoke of poisons in one section and poisons and instruments in another. Its main weakness was that it gave added legitimacy to the concept of quickening which meant that the woman herself or possibly a jury of matrons was to determine in a traditional, unscientific manner whether or not foetal life was present. Doctors therefore attacked the concept of quickening, not because they were necessarily better qualified than ordinary women to determine how far gestation had progressed but because to accept the inclusion of the notion of quickening on the statute books would signify that in some medical matters the word of the patient had as much legal weight as that of the doctor.[96]

Doctors asserted that 'quickening' only referred to the woman's sensation of the foetus moving but that in fact the vitality of the embryo was present from the moment of conception. All attempts at any point in the process of gestation to induce miscarriage were therefore equally culpable.

One of the first so to criticize the 1803 law was John Burns who declared in 1807 that

> many people at least pretend to view attempts to excite abortion as different from murder, upon the principle that the embryo is not possessed of life, in the common acceptance of the word. It undoubtedly can neither think nor act; but upon the same reasoning, we should conclude it to be innocent to kill the child in the birth.[97]

In 1815, Bartley declared only the 'uninformed and ignorant' assumed that there was no life in the embryo;[98] in 1816 Male asserted that it was 'probable' that the foetus was animated from the moment of conception;[99] in 1820 Dr Hutchinson told his students that though it was difficult to determine if a woman were pregnant the doctor had to consider a foetus 'alive' until it was expulsed.[100] Smith in 1821 and Paris and Fonblanque in 1823 all agreed that the law had only led to confusion by referring to 'quickening'.[101] In 1825 Beck and Dunlop went so far as to say that the ideas about quickening were positively pernicious: 'It may be said of them, with perfect truth, that their direct tendency has been to counten-ance rather than to encourage abortion, at least in the earlier stages of pregnancy.'[102] For these authors the foetus had to be alive or dead; since it was not expelled (as dead matter would be), it therefore was alive. If its movements were not sensed by the mother then that was due to a lack of consciousness on the part of the mother, not of the foetus. The laws were therefore subversive, declared Beck and Dunlop, by giving some credi-bility to the myth of quickening. 'They tempt to the perpetration of the same crime at one time which at another they punish with death'.[103] Charles Severn said much the same thing in 1831: 'the difference which the law makes in the nature of and punishment awarded to crimes involving the same degree of moral turpitude, is arbitrary and unfounded'.[104] In attacking the idea of either the mother or a jury of matrons deciding whether a woman was 'quick with child', Ryan lamented,

> The law of this Empire is extremely defective on abortion, for it abounds with the greatest absurdities. Its intention is humane and excellent, but it is based upon erroneous physiological principles. It enacts, for instance, that the embryo is not animated until after quickening, that is until half the period of uterogestation has lapsed, tho' the foetus is alive from the very moment of conception.[105]

Traill in 1836 noted that in France no legal line was drawn through the period of gestation, but 'The laws of Britain recognize this crime only after the period of *quickening*, on the false idea that then only life enters in the foetus.'[106] Finally, in 1837 Dr A. T. Thompson referred in the *Lancet* to the quickening as

> a singular instance of the difficulty of rooting out prejudice from the mind. . . . This distinction with respect to the periods in which criminal abortion is effected, demonstrates very strongly, the necessity of lawyers and statesmen consulting medical men, prior to framing Acts which involve physiological questions.[107]

Why were such strenuous attacks made by doctors on quickening? It was not just because the concept was scientifically untenable. Rather, as Thompson's reference made clear, doctors were intent on eliciting from lawyers the respect due to fellow professionals. The first decades of the nineteenth century witnessed a rash of texts on forensic medicine produced by medical men.[108] Many of our references to abortion have been taken from these very works because induction of miscarriage was a classic case in which medical and legal interests would cross. Of primary concern to doctors was the fear that in such contests their fledgling profession could be humiliated. Porter warned his medical students: 'A manifestation of ignorance on some important question . . . put to you in the witness box, might ruin your reputation, and, as far as your fortune is concerned, nullify all your other requirements.'[109] Such humiliations could be expected when concepts such as quickening, in being sanctioned by the law, placed the medical witness on unfamiliar terrain.

The trial of Charles Angus in the 1808 Lancaster summer assizes was a case in point. Angus was a Liverpool druggist whose wife had died a few years previously. Her half-sister, Margaret Burns, came to live in Angus's home to act as governess for his three children and, so it was later asserted, as his mistress. In March of 1808 Burns fell ill under suspicious circumstances and soon died. A coroner's examination was carried out and Angus subsequently charged with murder and with administering poisons with the intention of procuring abortion. In the trial which took place in September evidence was given by the servants of the Angus household that Burns slept with the master and was thought to be pregnant. Angus, for his part, was presented by the prosecution as having publicly defended the moral legitimacy of abortion: 'there is an easy method of doing it'. Abortion, he was reported as saying, 'may be occasioned with great safety'. A friend, Peter Charnely, testified that Angus dismissed moral arguments against abortion. 'I observed, that to do such a thing was a great sin – he replied, "the sin lay in taking away life, but not in preventing it".' Moreover, Angus had in his possession a variety of medical instruments and a supply of savin oil, the well-known abortifacient that some druggists refused to sell to women for fear of the use that they would make of it. The questions of whether or not Burns had been aborted, 'quick with child,' or was even pregnant could not be agreed upon by the medical experts. The judge in summing up the confused state of their testimony concluded that the jury was put in a quandary: 'With respect to the circumstances of the deceased having been with child, you are put into the place of deciding where doctors disagree'.[110] After five minutes' deliberation the jurors declared the defendant not guilty. In the pamphlet war waged by the medical witnesses after the trial they made it clear how unhappy they were with the current legislation which forced them, when in the witness box, to grapple with the issue of quickening which was foreign to their vocabulary.[111] To avoid the sort of public demonstrations of professional disarray demonstrated at the Angus trial doctors sought revisions in the law that would bring it into harmony with their own terminology.

The second reason for the doctors' concern with the notion of quickening was that they were not only suspicious of the idea of the state stepping in to legislate on physiological matters;

they were also in the process of building up arguments against the idea that the patient could dictate the tactics to be adopted in a difficult pregnancy. The first modern English text of professional duties, Percival's *Medical Ethics*, appeared in the same year as the 1803 abortion law.[112] The subject of abortion found a key place in this text and all similar works in the following decades. A perusal of these studies' discussions of abortions and Caesarians reveals that though the issues were lumped together as problems of medical ethics they were in fact treated as problems of medical etiquette.[113] A doctor's decision to induce an abortion, for example, would be justified primarily on the basis of whether or not his colleagues had been consulted. Though doctors might differ in their attitudes towards abortion the writers of these texts repeatedly reminded them that their first concern had to be for the well-being of the profession. In making major decisions subject to agreement of fellow professionals one could ensure that colleague control replaced client control.[114] The concept of quickening was perhaps the best example of the patient having some power – that is to say, the power of determining if vitality were present – and it necessarily had to be sacrificed to practitioners who asserted that they alone could make such decisions.

The third and final point to be made about English doctors' attack on quickening is that it was based on their conviction that the concept was scientifically meaningless. They presented themselves as attempting to raise medical care above the particular interests of specific clients and beyond the reach of traditional prejudices. But their attempt to deal with abortion as merely one problem within the confines of a detached, objective medical science was undermined by the contradictory statements they made about the vitality of embryonic life. Whatever one might think of French Catholic physicians' condemnations of both criminal and therapeutic abortion, one has at least to recognize the consistency of their arguments. In contrast English doctors vaunted a foetal vitality when condemning the notion of quickening which they tended to dismiss when discussing therapeutic abortion.

The year 1837 in which Dr A. T. Thompson called for lawyers and statesmen to consult doctors when drawing up laws pertaining to medical matters did indeed see the law brought into line with the interests of the profession. The 1828 Act had removed some of the confusions of the 1803 statute by referring to the use of instruments as well as poisons, both before and after quickening. The Offences Against the Person Act of 1837 finally abolished the concept of quickening.[115] Ryan in 1841 and Radford in 1848 applauded the fact that the law was now based on the findings of physiology. But was it? The concept of quickening was legally obliterated and along with it the idea that the woman had some legal power of determining whether foetal life existed or not. Gone too was the 'jury of matrons' – Bracken's 'old doting women' – on occasion called in on abortion cases in the past, though Radford complained that they were still empowered to determine if a murderess under sentence of death were pregnant.[116] But no new physiological findings were actually incorporated in the new law. The issue of vitality was skirted altogether by holding culpable anyone who with *intent* to commit abortion employed drugs or instruments on *any* woman. In short, the woman did not even have to be pregnant. This suggests that though the revisions to the abortion law came in part in response to medical lobbying, the refining and clarification of the statutes obviously also followed an inherent legal logic that simplified their exercise.[117] Nevertheless the new statute was presented by doctors and did seem to be part of a successful campaign waged, if not to incorporate new medical views, at least to eliminate traditional concepts in the law to which the profession objected.[118]

At the start of this chapter it was asked why the abortion laws emerged when they did. Did they represent a new concern for the protection of foetal life or a new desire to discipline women's childbearing? One must conclude that though elements of both concerns existed they do not provide a full explanation for the passage of the new statutes. The abortion law that emerged in 1803 was an unexpected consequence of a long campaign by humanitarians to abolish the law on infanticide. The abortion law as it emerged from the revisions of 1828 and 1837 was a product on the one hand of lawyers, to simplify its working, and on the other of medical men, to purge the statute book of all references to quickening. This latter change meant that vitality was now taken to be present from the moment of conception. As a consequence actions traditionally not subjected to prosecution were now declared to be criminal although in practice only when carried out by non-medical personnel. No doctor acting in consultation with his colleagues was ever prosecuted for abortion. Doctors had accomplished the remarkable feat of creating a taboo which they alone could freely violate.

Control over fertility is a basic aspect of family life. The abortion laws were important, not because they necessarily made recourse to inducement of miscarriage any less likely, but because they signalled the intention of the medical and legal professions to intervene in matters of fertility control. A corollary of the professionals' new power would ultimately be a decline in women's rights to limit their pregnancies. Foucault and Donzelot have asserted that in late eighteenth- and early nineteenth-century France it was the growth of fears and fantasies concerning sexuality which gave rise to an obsessive desire on the part of professionals to control sexual behaviour.[119] The investigation of the abortion laws of early nineteenth-century England reveals that such desires for control did indeed exist but that they emerged from more mundane interests. The shift in public attitudes towards embryonic life would later be attributed to religious pre-occupations with the sanctity of foetal life, to new scientific appreciations of the process of gestation, and to a growing emotional and sentimental concern for the child. But significant, also, were the pragmatic concerns and professional interests of lawyers and doctors seeking to implement laws that would best serve their needs.

The 1803 statute obviously did not end women's recourse to abortion. Women's responses to the law varied from resistance, to accommodation, to protest.[120] But in some ways 1803 did mark a turning-point. It has been noted that traditional ideas concerning the process of procreation were in the eighteenth century increasingly satirized and castigated by the enlightened and the respectable, and in this chapter we have seen how one aspect of this clash of sexual cultures ultimately concluded. The criminalization of a crucial form of fertility control – abortion – signalled more emphatically than could any other action the erosion of the traditional reproductive rituals of early modern England.

Conclusion

This book began by comparing what historians and cultural anthropologists had to say about pre-industrial societies' interest in and ability to control reproduction. Various views have been published: for instance, that earlier generations – because they had high fertility rates – were indifferent to the problems posed by childbearing; and that medical historians who did note the vast range of rules, regulations, charms and herbal remedies employed by couples for the purposes of effecting conception and gestation concluded that they did not warrant serious investigation because they did not 'work'; but also that there is abundant evidence to indicate that well before 1800 control of conceptions was both thinkable and possible.

There has been an obvious but unfounded assumption that because the fertility of seventeenth- and eighteenth-century couples was high they must have lacked both an interest in and an ability to lower it. However, simple restriction of family size is not the sole criterion of a society's concern with controlling conceptions. Other cultures, studied by anthropologists, have employed a variety of fertility-affecting agents for purposes that are often quite foreign to the western, modern mind. As regards the second assertion, concerning the ineffectiveness of traditional contraceptives and abortifacients, anthropologists have had further useful insights to offer. They suggest that setting aside the possible physiological effects of such remedies it must be remembered that they can often be said to 'work' on a psychological level inasmuch as they are part of a popular model of physiology in which men and women are regarded as having some control over fertility. It is evident that via a variety

145

of traditional methods employed either to promote or restrict fertility ordinary English men and women did feel that they understood and participated in the process of conception. Although in such a short work it has not been possible to analyse and satisfactorily explain every aspect of the early modern discussion of procreation anthropological insights do cast a fresh light on traditional English attitudes towards sexuality, fertility, contraception and abortion.

In chapter one we sought to show that sexual pleasure and procreation were linked in the popular mind by a traditional Galenic model of physiology. Women's sexuality (according to this model) was acknowledged and valued. Despite the claims of some historians that it was only in the eighteenth century that the pleasure principle emerged, we discovered that as a consequence of the elaboration of more sophisticated models of reproduction in the later 1700s the rights of women to sexual pleasure were not enhanced but eroded. Medical scientists were, of course, not the only ones seeking in the eighteenth century to redefine sex roles. This study does not argue that doctors alone created the new ideal of female sexual passivity. Given the limited readership of their works their impact could not have been, by itself, decisive; they influenced and were influenced by other participants in the discussion. Nevertheless, because of their expertise in physiology, doctors clearly were an important element in the reappraisal of female sexual needs.

In the earlier period women's sexuality was perceived as important because it was directly related to their fertility. The belief that their pleasure was necessary to ensure conception implied that procreation could be controlled.

Having argued in chapter one that traditional medical beliefs held that men and women could exert some control over procreation we turned, in chapter two, to examine the ways in which earlier generations sought to determine the course of conceptions, pregnancies and births. Such tactics were, because of the great social emphasis placed on childbearing, often employed for the purposes of promoting fertility. Of the countless injunctions made by writers since 1500 to increase and multiply, Shakespeare's are, to modern readers, perhaps the most familiar.

Look in thy glass, and tell the face thou viewest
Now is the time that face should form another;

Whose fresh repair if now thou not renewest,
Thou dost beguile the world, unbless some mother.
For where is she so fair whose uneared womb
Disdains the tillage of thy husbandry?
Or who is he so fond will be the tomb
Of his self-love, to stop posterity?

Thou art thy mother's glass, and she in thee
Calls back the lovely April of her prime:
So though through windows of thine age shalt see,
Despite of wrinkles, this thy golden time.
But if thou live, remembered not to be,
Die single, and thine image dies with thee.[1]

Less well known and therefore subject to closer analysis were the enormous number of herbals, midwifery texts, chapbooks and receipt books that contained a pot-pourri of information on how conceptions could be best assured and pregnancies protected. It was this sort of power over reproduction that bulked largest in the early modern writings on sexuality.

Many of the same taboos and herbal potions employed to *promote* fertility were also used to restrict it. The debate over the regulation of reproduction provided, in even its most hardened attacks on contraception, proof of the 'thinkability' of such practices. The various methods employed to limit births, and the range of cultural factors which could affect the choice of contraceptive method – age of mother, nursing pattern, physiological beliefs and so on – were examined in chapter three. Some worked; some did not. The important point made in this chapter was that recourse to such methods indicated that earlier generations did on occasion seek to space or limit births and were not indifferent to the real dangers repeated pregnancies could pose to the health and happiness of the household.[2]

In earlier times abortion played an important, though as yet little-recognized, role in fertility control, and the motives of women and the methods they employed were analysed in chapter four. It was not so much the act itself as the question of who aborted, when, and why, that preoccupied the community. The concept of quickening made recourse to abortion possibly more thinkable for past generations. In studying abortion beliefs it is possible to glimpse aspects of a separate female sexual culture that supports the independence and autonomy of women from medical men, moralists and spouses.[3]

147

In order to understand why women's reproductive behaviour appeared to be subjected to greater public scrutiny at the end of the eighteenth century, chapter five provided an account of the early religious, medical and legal discussions of abortion. The 1803 statute was in the first instance a result of the campaign for the reform of the infanticide law. But in making the law on infanticide more lenient the 1803 statute made abortion before quickening a crime. More rather than less legal interference in childbearing inevitably ensued.

The 1803 abortion act did not, however, so much concern the foetus as it did the mother, and this book has only followed the law through its 1828 and 1837 revisions. Only in the course of its nineteenth-century revisions would the statute become the instrument pro-natalists sought. Analysis revealed that they reflected the medical profession's hostility to the original acts' placing the concept of quickening on the statute books. The early abortion laws were more a consequence of the medical and legal professions' attempts to serve their own interests than to affect directly fertility. The laws, nevertheless, provided the basis for a new policing of the fertility of the lower orders; the old world in which sexual activities were held in check by the moral coercion of the community was being replaced by a new society in which laws were passed by one class and sex for the policing of another.

Is it possible to gauge the result of the assaults on the older beliefs concerning procreation and the emergence of the new biomedical model? A common assumption is that 'modernization' – industrialization, urbanization, education, the decline of old myths and taboos, the rise of secular values, and the emergence of the professions – made fertility control both thinkable and possible. Most histories of birth control begin in the late eighteenth century when such modernization is said to have begun. But the inherent weakness of such an approach is the fact that fertility in England did not decline after 1750; rather it rose and continued at a high level until the mid-nineteenth century. Why? In part because the process of modernization in the first place created a new demand for child labour and in the second place undermined many of the traditional restraints on fertility.[4] Industrialization and urbanization, in relaxing the controls on marriage previously exerted by apprenticeship contracts and rural inheritance customs, allowed more people to marry and to marry earlier;

the factory work of women, in making extended breastfeeding more difficult, deprived them of the protection of post-partum amenorrhoea; the rise of secular values weakened the old patterns of sexual abstinence; the emergence of the medical profession eroded traditional reliances on herbal potions; and the courts, in making abortion before quickening a crime, closed off a traditional means of fertility control. It is, of course, difficult to determine quantitatively the impact of each of these changes, but that is not, in any event, the purpose of this study. This book was written to demonstrate simply the ingenuity and perseverance with which men and women of earlier generations sought to control fertility.

The interpretation of the past that this book has been questioning holds that until the eighteenth or nineteenth century the idea and practice of controlling fertility were not found in England. It would be anachronistic to argue that prior to 1750 modern birth control methods were being employed for the twentieth-century purpose of 'family planning': both the notion that attitudes towards fertility regulation massively changed at some decisive moment and the notion that such attitudes never changed are equally wrongheaded. The industrialized, urbanized England of the nineteenth century differed so fundamentally from the largely rural, communal England that we have been examining that it is clearly impossible to suggest that there was some simple linear increase or decrease in the concern for controlling conceptions.

There was no single coherent system of fertility regulation in past times. This study has sought simply to examine the variety of forms reproductive regulation might take. Its outline of the range of controls has been necessarily impressionistic, but it has nevertheless revealed the variety of options open to couples in early modern England. And in looking closely at the issue of reproductive control it has also sought to uncover many of the attitudes, experiences and values of a culture that would otherwise have remained obscure. The conceiving and bearing of children is one of the most fascinating experiences in which we can ever become involved; each and every society attempts by its own particular means and for its own particular purposes to control the process, and in so doing reveals key concerns and convictions.

What has our investigation of beliefs concerning repro-duction told us about earlier generations? It has revealed that

149

they were neither automata nor simply ignorant, abject victims of biological forces. Childbearing was, of course, painful and fraught with danger, but that did not mean that men and women when confronted by it were paralysed by fear. On the contrary, just because the conceiving and bearing of children was so important previous generations elaborated a remarkable range of strategies to deal with each stage of the procreative process. It is difficult in fact not to think that we today have a much more impoverished sense of our powers when contemplating parenthood. This is in part because in some ways we have developed a rigid, mechanical view of reproduction. Parents in the past perceived it as mutable – conditioned by diet, exercise, potions and charms. They believed that nature and culture interacted and that their fertility was accordingly their own social creation.

Notes

Introduction

[1] Edward Shorter, *The Making of the Modern Family* (New York: Basic Books, 1975).

[2] David Hunt, *Parents and Children in History: the psychology of family life in early modern France* (New York: Basic Books, 1970), 82–3.

[3] John Knodel and Etienne van de Walle, 'Lessons from the past: policy implications of historical fertility studies', *Population and Development Review*, 5 (1979), 227.

[4] Laurel Thatcher Ulrich, *Good Wives: Image and reality in the lives of women in northern New England, 1650–1750* (New York: Knopf, 1982), 159.

[5] E. P. Thompson, 'Eighteenth-century English society: class struggle without class', *Social History*, 3 (1978), 157–8.

[6] Lawrence Stone, *The Family, Sex, and Marriage in England, 1500–1800* (New York: Harper & Row, 1977; Harmondsworth: Penguin, 1979), 234, 415, 416.

[7] Edward Shorter, *A History of Women's Bodies* (New York: Basic Books, 1982), 3.

[8] See for example Clellan S. Ford, *A Comparative Study of Human Reproduction* (New Haven: Yale Publications in Anthropology, no. 32, 1945); F. Lorimer, *Culture and Human Fertility* (New York: UNESCO, 1954); Geoffrey Hawthorn, *The Sociology of Fertility* (London: Macmillan, 1970).

[9] Bronislow Malinowski, *Sex, Culture, and Myth* (London: Dell, 2nd edn 1967), 74; and see also *Sex and Repression in Savage Society* (London: Routledge & Kegan Paul, 1960).

[10] Anthropology and history have been successfully wedded in such works as Keith Thomas, *Religion and the Decline of Magic: Studies in popular beliefs in sixteenth- and seventeenth-century England* (Harmondsworth: Penguin, 1971) and Alan Macfarlane, *The Family Life*

of Ralph Josselin: A seventeenth-century clergyman (Cambridge: Cambridge University Press, 1970). Like Thomas and Macfarlane I am adopting the approach of a particular school of anthropology. Some anthropologists are hostile to such attempts at collaboration, arguing that civilized and primitive societies are so qualitatively different that no meaningful comparisons can be drawn between their economic, political or cultural patterns.

[11] Bernice Kaplan (ed.), *Anthropological Studies of Human Fertility* (Detroit: Wayne State University Press, 1976).

[12] See for example Warren M. Hern, 'Knowledge and use of herbal contraceptives in a Peruvian Amazon village', *Human Organization*, 35 (1976), 9–20.

[13] See for example George S. Masnick and Solomon H. Katz, 'Adaptive childbearing in a northern slope Eskimo community', in Kaplan, *Studies*, 37–58; M. C. Goldstein, 'New perspectives on Tibetan fertility and population decline', *American Ethnologist*, 8 (1981), 721 ff.

[14] On the concept of 'natural fertility' see Louis Henry, 'Fondements théoriques des mesures de la fécondité naturelle', *Revue de l'Institut International de Statistique*, 21 (1953), 135–51; *Anciennes familles genèvoises: études démographiques: 16e–20e siècles* (Paris: Presses Universitaires de France, 1956); 'Some data on natural fertility', *Eugenics Quarterly*, 8 (1961), 81–91; 'Concepts actuels et résultats empiriques sur la fécondité naturelle', in H. Leridon and J. Menken (eds), *Natural Fertility: Patterns and determinants of natural fertility* (Liège: Ordina, 1979). On anthropologists' views see Moni Nag, *Factors Affecting Human Fertility in Nonindustrial Societies: A cross cultural study* (New Haven: Yale University Publications in Anthropology, no. 66, 1962); Carol P. MacCormack (ed.), *Ethnography of Fertility and Birth* (New York: Academic Press, 1982), 1–4.

[15] See R. Lesthaeghe, 'On the social control of human reproduction', *Population and Development Review*, 6 (1980), 527–48.

[16] Patricia James, *Population Malthus: His life and times* (London: Routledge & Kegan Paul, 1979).

[17] See for example John W. M. Whiting, 'Effects of climate on certain cultural practices', in Ward E. Goodenough (ed.), *Explorations in Cultural Anthropology* (New York: McGraw-Hill, 1964), 511–44; Susan B. Hanley, 'The influence of economic and social variables on marriage and fertility in eighteenth- and nineteenth-century Japanese villages', in R. D. Lee (ed.), *Population Patterns in the Past* (New York: Academic Press, 1977), 165–200; Raymond Firth, *We, The Tikopia* (London: Allen & Unwin, 1936); W. D. Borrie, Raymond Firth, James Spillius, 'The population of Tikopia, 1929 and 1952', *Population Studies*, 10 (1956–7), 229–52; J. C. Caldwell and P. Caldwell, 'The function of child spacing in traditional societies and the direction of change', in H. J. Page and R. Lesthaeghe (eds), *Child Spacing in Tropical Africa: Traditions and change* (Toronto: Academic Press, 1981), 74–91; P. Cantrelle and B. Ferry,

'Approche de la fécondité naturelle dans les populations contemporaines', in H. Leridon and J. Menken (eds), *Natural Fertility: Patterns and determinants of natural fertility* (Liège: Ordina, 1979); E. Weis and A. A. Udo, 'The Calabar rural maternal and child health/family planning project', *Studies in Family Planning*, 12 (1981), 47–57.

[18] Norman E. Himes, *Medical History of Contraception* (Baltimore: Williams & Wilkins, 1936), 170–83; Shorter, *Women's Bodies*, 77–9.

[19] The Tully River aborigines have drawn so much attention because they are almost unique among primitive cultures in not appearing to recognize either biological paternity or maternity. See Ashley Montagu, *Coming into Being Among the Australian Aborigines: A study of the procreative beliefs of the native tribes of Australia* (London: Routledge & Kegan Paul, 2nd edn 1974), 326–34; Melford E. Spiro, 'Virgin births, parthenogenesis, and physiological paternity: an essay in cultural interpretation', *Man*, 3 (1968), 242–61; Sir Edmund Leach, *Genesis as Myth and Other Essays* (London: Cape, 1969).

[20] Thomas, *Religion*, 301–35.

[21] See for example George Devereux, *Abortion in Primitive Society* (New York: International, 2nd edn 1976).

[22] Kingsley Davis and Judith Blake, 'Social structure and fertility: an analytical framework', *Economic Development and Cultural Change*, 4 (1955), 211–35.

[23] M. Morokvasic, 'Sexuality and control of procreation', in K. Young *et al.* (eds), *Of Marriage and the Market* (London: CSE Books, 1981), 139.

[24] Mernissi cited in Barbara Rogers, *The Domestication of Women: Discrimination in developing societies* (London: Tavistock Publications, 1981), 114.

[25] Jane F. Collier in reviewing Karen P. Paige and Jeffrey M. Paige, *The Politics of Reproductive Rituals* (Berkeley: University of California Press, 1981) points out the work's failure to discriminate between male and female desires in reproduction, and comments: 'In all societies, the motives people attribute to women are related to the motives they attribute to men, but seldom are they identical'. *Science*, 215 (1982), 1230. For a selection of essays touching on the same theme see Carol MacCormack and Marilyn Strathern (eds), *Nature, Culture, and Gender* (Cambridge: Cambridge University Press, 1980).

[26] Steven Polgar, 'Population history and population policies from an anthropological perspective', *Current Anthropology*, 13 (1972), 203–11; J. C. Caldwell and P. Caldwell, 'The role of marital sexual abstinence in determining fertility: A study of the Yoruba in Nigeria', *Population Studies*, 31 (1977), 193–213; H. Page and R. Lesthaeghe, *Child Spacing in Tropical Africa* (Toronto: Academic Press, 1979). On the prolonging of breastfeeding in pre-industrial societies to delay the next pregnancy see J. Knodel, 'Lessons from the past: Policy implications of historical fertility studies', *Population and Development Review* 5 (1979), 1–20;

'Espacement des naissances et planification familiale: une critique de la méthode Dupâquier-Lachiver,' *Annales Economies, Sociétés, Civilisations,* 36 (1981), 473–88; J. Dupâquier and M. Lachiver, 'Du contresens à l'illusion technique', *Annales Economies, Sociétés, Civilisations,* 36 (1981), 489–95; M. Singarimbum and C. Manning, 'Breast feeding, amenorrhoea and abstinence in a Javanese Village: A case study of Mojolama', *Studies in Family Planning,* 7 (1976), 175–80.

[27] On the issue of ignorance of birth control methods in 'advanced societies' see Lee Rainwater, *And the Poor Get Children: Sex, contraceptives and family planning in the working classes* (Chicago: Quadrangle, 1960); Shirley M. Johnson and Loudell F. Snow, 'Assessment of reproductive knowledge in an inner city clinic', *Social Science and Medicine,* 16 (1982), 1657–62.

[28] Gyorgy T. Acsadi, 'Traditional birth control methods in Yorubaland', in J. F. Marshal and S. Polgar (eds), *Culture, Natality, and Family Planning* (Chapel Hill: University of North Carolina Press, 1976), 126–55.

[29] See for example MacCormack, *Ethnography,* 65–6; Mary-Jo Delvecchio Good, 'Of blood and babies: the relationship of popular Islamic physiology to fertility', *Social Science and Medicine,* 14B (1980), 147–56.

[30] Rogers, *Domestication,* 111.

[31] T. H. Hollingsworth, *Historical Demography* (London: Hodder & Stoughton, 1969); Thomas McKeown, *The Modern Rise of Population* (London: Edward Arnold, 1976).

[32] E. A. Wrigley and R. S. Schofield, *The Population History of England 1541–1871* (London: Edward Arnold, 1981), 230.

[33] E. A. Wrigley, 'Family limitation in pre-industrial England', *Economic History Review,* 19 (1966), 82–109; David Levine, *Family Formation in an Age of Nascent Capitalism* (New York: Academic Press, 1977), 64; David Levine and Keith Wrightson, *Poverty and Piety in an English Village: Terling, 1525–1700* (New York: Academic Press, 1979), 49–56, 63 ff.; Keith Wrightson, *English Society, 1580–1680* (London: Hutchinson, 1982), 105; Daniel Scott Smith in Lee, *Population,* 33–7.

[34] M. W. Flinn, *The European Demographic System* (Baltimore: Johns Hopkins University Press, 1981), 84; and see also Flinn's review of Wrigley and Schofield in the *Economic History Review,* 25 (1982), 443–57.

[35] Shorter, *Modern Family,* 56–65.

[36] Stone, *Family,* 324–36.

[37] Wrightson, *English Society,* 89–104.

[38] Michael MacDonald, *Mystical Bedlam: Madness, anxiety, and healing in seventeenth-century England* (Cambridge: Cambridge University Press, 1981), 98–105. See also Alan Macfarlane, *The Family Life of Ralph Josselin,* 106–10; Peter Laslett, *The World We Have Lost* (London: Methuen, 3rd edn 1983), 22.

[39] MacDonald, *Mystical Bedlam*, 80 ff., 259–60.

[40] Shorter, *Modern Family*, 169–75; Stone, *Family*, 161–79, 194–5. See also Lloyd de Mause (ed.), *History of Childhood* (New York: Harper & Row, 1974); Ivy Pinchbeck and Margaret Hewitt, *Children in English Society*, Volume I; *From Tudor Times to the Eighteenth Century* (London: Routledge & Kegan Paul, 1969), 7–22.

[41] Wrightson, *English Society*, 104–18; B. A. Hanawalt, 'Child rearing among the lower classes of late medieval England', *Journal of Interdisciplinary History*, 8 (1977), 1–22.

[42] Natalie Z. Davis, 'The possibilities of the past', *Journal of Interdisciplinary History*, 12 (1981), 267–76.

[43] The studies that most closely approximate to what this work seeks to do have dealt with French families. See for example Emmanuel Le Roy Ladurie, *Montaillou* (New York: Pantheon, 1980; Harmondsworth: Penguin, 1980); Natalie Z. Davis, *Society and Culture in Early Modern France* (Stanford: Stanford University Press, 1975); Jacques Gélis *et al.*, *Entrer dans la vie: naissances et enfances dans la France traditionnelle* (Paris: Gallimard, 1978); Jean-Louis Flandrin, *Les amours paysannes, XVIe–XIXe siècles* (Paris: Gallimard, 1975). See also Randolph Trumbach, 'London's Sodomites: Homosexual behavior and western culture in the eighteenth century', *Journal of Social History*, 11 (1977), 1–33.

1 *The pleasures of procreation*

[1] Edward Shorter, *A History of Women's Bodies* (New York: Basic Books, 1982), 16.

[2] See for example Clifford Geertz, *The Interpretation of Cultures* (New York: Basic Books, 1973).

[3] Everard Home, 'An account of the dissection of an hermaphrodite dog', *Philosophical Transactions of the Royal Society* (1799), 162, and see also F. N. L. Poynter, 'Hunter, Spallanzani, and the history of artificial insemination', in L. G. Stevenson and R. P. Multhauf, *Medicine, Science and Culture: Historical essays in honor of Oswei Temkin* (Baltimore: Johns Hopkins University Press, 1968).

[4] Randolph Trumbach, *The Rise of the Egalitarian Family: Aristocratic kinship and domestic relations in eighteenth-century England* (New York: Academic Press, 1978); Lawrence Stone, *The Family, Sex and Marriage in England, 1500–1800* (New York: Harper & Row, 1977; Harmondsworth: Penguin, 1979); Edward Shorter, *The Making of the Modern Family* (New York: Harper & Row, 1976). For a more sensitive view of the eighteenth century see Roy Porter, 'Mixed feelings: the enlightenment and sexuality in eighteenth-century Britain', in P. G. Boucé (ed.), *Sexuality in Eighteenth-Century England* (Manchester: Manchester University Press, 1982), 1–27.

[5] On the notions of high and low cultures see Natalie Z. Davis, *Society and Culture in Sixteenth-Century France* (Stanford: Stanford University Press, 1975); Peter Burke, *Popular Culture in Early Modern Europe* (London: Temple Smith, 1978); Christopher Hill, *The World Turned Upside Down: Radical ideas during the English Revolution* (London: Temple Smith, 1972).

[6] See Edmund S. Morgan, 'The Puritans and sex', *New England Quarterly*, 15 (1942), 591–607; Edmund Leites, 'The duty to desire: love, friendship, and sexuality in some Puritan theories of marriage', *Journal of Social History*, 15 (1982), 383–408; W. and M. Haller, 'The Puritan art of love', *Huntingdon Library Quarterly*, 5 (1941–2), 235–72; M. Todd, 'Humanists, Puritans and the spiritualized household', *Church History*, 49 (1980), 18–34.

[7] William Gouge, *Of Domesticall Duties: Eight Treatises* (London: Haviland, 1622), 223.

[8] Gataker cited in James T. Johnson, 'English Puritan thought on the ends of marriage', *Church History*, 38 (1969), 430.

[9] On French views of sexuality see Pierre Darmon, *Le Mythe de la procréation à l'âge baroque* (Paris: Pauvret, 1977).

[10] Aristotle, *De Partibus Animalium I and De Generatione Animalium I*, tr. D. M. Balme (Oxford: Clarendon, 1972), 48.

[11] See for example Anthony Preus, 'Science and philosophy in Aristotle's Generation of Animals', *Journal of the History of Biology*, 3 (1970), 1–52.

[12] Cited in Howard B. Adelman, *Marcello Malpighi and the Evolution of Embryology* (Ithaca: Cornell University Press, 1966), II, 737.

[13] Anthony Preus, 'Galen's criticisms of Aristotle's conception theory', *Journal of the History of Biology*, 10 (1977), 65–85. On hostility to the Galenic view that women produced seed see M. Anthony Hewson, *Giles of Rome and the Medieval Theory of Conception* (London: Athlone, 1975).

[14] On the semence theory in the Middle Ages see Helen R. Lemay, 'Human sexuality in twelfth through fifteenth century scientific writings', in Verne Bullough and James Brundage (eds), *Sexual Practices and the Medieval Church* (Buffalo: Prometheus, 1982), 187–203; for the Renaissance see Ian Maclean, *The Renaissance Notion of Women* (Cambridge: Cambridge University Press, 1980), 28–33; for sixteenth-century England see Levine Lemnie, *The Touchstone of Complexions*, tr. Thomas Newton (London: Barth, 1581), 108; Thomas Cogan, *The Haven of Health* (London: Midleton, 1584), 245.

[15] Thomas Raynald, *The Birth of Man-Kinde* (London: A.H., 1634), 41; see also Helkiah Crooke, *A Description of the Body of Man* (London: Taggard, 1618), 202, 216, 261, 295.

[16] Nathaniel Highmore, *The History of Generation* (London: John Martin, 1651), 85.

[17] S. Wilkins (ed.), *Sir Thomas Browne's Works* (London: Pickering, 1835), III, 345.

[18] *The Works of William Harvey*, tr. Robert Willis (London: Sydenham Society, 1965), 294.

[19] A Physician [Nicolas Venette], *Conjugal Love Reveal'd* (London: Hinton, 1720), 37; John Maubray, *The Female Physician* (London: Holland, 1724), 20; and see also Henry Bracken, *The Midwife's Companion* (London: J. Clarke, 1737), 12. On the changing presentation of conception compare *Aristotle's Masterpiece* (London: J. How, 1690), 10, to *The Works of Aristotle* (Derby: Richardson, 1840?), 15. On the semence view in France see the French equivalent of *Aristotle's Masterpiece*, the anonymous *Les admirables secrets d'Albert le Grand* (Cologne, 1722), 2.

[20] M*** [Michel Procope-Couteau], *L'Art de faire garçons ou nouveau tableau de l'amour conjugal* (Montpellier: Maugiron, 2nd edn 1760), 25.

[21] For one woman's acknowledgement of her and her husband's 'inordinate love, and the great delectation they each had in using the other' see the fourteenth-century work, *The Book of Margery Kemp* (New York: Devin-Adair, 1944), 6; see also on the earlier period Edith Whitehurst Williams, 'What's so new about the sexual revolution?', *Texas Quarterly*, 18 (1975), 46–55.

[22] But for the argument that Venette best captured the late seventeenth-century portrayal of sexuality see the stimulating introduction by Roy Porter (ed.), Nicolas Venette, *The Mysteries of Conjugal Love Revealed* (London: Junction Books, forthcoming).

[23] See Otho T. Beall, '*Aristotle's Masterpiece* in America: a landmark in the folklore of medicine', *William and Mary Quarterly*, 20 (1963), 207–22; Verne Bullough, 'An early American sex manual: or Aristotle who?', *Early American Literature*, 7 (1973), 236–46; Janet Blackman, 'Popular theories of generation', in John Woodward and David Richards (eds), *Health Care and Popular Medicine in Nineteenth-Century England* (London: Croom Helm, 1977).

[24] *Aristotle's Masterpiece* (1690), 2. Similarly, Johannes Johnstonus warned in *An History of the Wonderful Things of Nature* (London: John Streater, 1657), 326–7, that the unexpended 'seed' of widows and virgins caused melancholy.

[25] *Aristotle's Masterpiece* (1690), 98; see also *Aristotle's Compleat Masterpiece* (London: Booksellers, 1749), 16.

[26] Bracken, *Companion*, 10.

[27] E. Sibly, *The Medical Mirror or Treatise on the Impregnation of the Human Female* (London: 1794), 23.

[28] Venette, *Conjugal Love*, 161; *Aristotle's Masterpiece* (1690), 23–4; Johnstonus, *History*, 30. On the continent Agrippa of Nettesheim went so far as to twist Galen's theory to assert that children were products of the female seed alone. 'It is the seed of woman alone, as Galen and

Avicenna say, that is the matter and nutriment of the fetus, least of all the man's which enters into the woman as an accident into the substance'. Cited in Arlene Miller Guinsburg, 'The counterthrust to sixteenth-century misogyny: the work of Agrippa and Paracelsus', *Historical Reflections/Réflexions historiques*, 8 (1981), 3–28.

[29] Lazarus Riverius *et al.*, *The Practice of Physick* (London: Cole, 1658), 503.

[30] James McMath, *The Expert Midwife* (Edinburgh: Mosman, 1694), 3.

[31] Bracken, *Companion*, 10; Sibly, *Mirror*, 17.

[32] James Guillemeau cited in Audrey Eccles, *Obstetrics and Gynaecology in Tudor and Stuart England* (London: Croom Helm, 1982), 29. See also Robert H. Michel, 'English attitudes towards women, 1640–1700', *Canadian Journal of History*, 13 (1978), 43–4.

[33] Jane Sharp, *The Compleat Midwife's Companion: or the art of midwifery improved* (London: Marshall, 2nd edn 1725), 109; and see also the comments of a recent historian of seventeenth-century chapbooks: 'Certainly, the whole tenor of the merry books conveys that seventeenth-century women enjoyed their own sexuality and were expected to enjoy it.' Margaret Spufford, *Small Books and Pleasant Histories: Popular fiction and its readership in seventeenth-century England* (London: Methuen, 1981), 63.

[34] P. Barrough, *The Method of Physick* (London: Vautroullier, 1583), 157.

[35] Riverius, *Physick*, 503.

[36] Nicholas Culpeper, *A Directory for Midwives* (London: Peter Cole, 1660), 70.

[37] John Sadler, *The Sick Woman's Private Looking Glass* (Norwood, N. J., W. J. Johnson, 1977, first edn 1656), 108–9.

[38] Samuel Farr, *Elements of Medical Jurisprudence* (London: Callow, 2nd edn 1815), 46; and for similar views see *Aristotle's Last Legacy* (London: Butterbox, 1789), 363, and *Aristotle's Compleat and Experienced Midwife* (London: Booksellers, 1700), 132.

[39] John Pechey, *The Compleat Midwife's Practice Enlarged* (London: Rhodes, 1694), 243.

[40] John Bulwer, *Anthrometamorphosis: Man Transformed; or the Artificial Changeling* (London: Hardesty, 1650), 213.

[41] Sharp, *Midwife*, 36.

[42] See Eccles cited above in footnote 32 and Jacques Roger, *Les sciences de la vie dans la pensée française du XVIIIᵉ siècle* (Paris: Colin, 1963).

[43] Adelman, *Malpighi*, II, 733–77.

[44] Harvey, *Works*, 362.

[45] Adelman, *Malpighi*, II, 861.

[46] For overviews see Elizabeth B. Gasking, *Investigations into Generation 1651–1828* (Baltimore: Johns Hopkins University Press,

1967), Charles W. Bodemer, 'Embryological thought in seventeenth century England', in Lester S. King (ed.), *Medical Investigations in Seventeenth Century England* (Los Angeles: University of California Press, 1968), 1–25; Joseph Needham, *A History of Embryology* (New York: Abelard-Schuman, 1959), 115–230.

[47] Helen Brock informs me that a claim can be made that W. Cruikshank discovered the egg as early as 1778 and reported it in the *Philosophical Transactions* in 1797. See also Needham, *History*, 217.

[48] John Case, *The Angelical Guide* (London: Dawkes, 1697), 53; Joseph Blondel, *The Strength of Imagination in Pregnant Women Examin'd* (London: J. Peele, 1727), 42; Alexander Hamilton, *A Treatise on Midwifery* (London: John Murray, 1781), 40; William Cullen (ed.), *First Lines of Physiology by the Celebrated Baron Albertus Haller* (Edinburgh: Elliot, 1786), II, 206–8; and see also A Physician, *A Rational Account of the Natural Weaknesses of Women* (London, n.p., 1727), 62.

[49] Although for the purposes of this study it is not especially important it should be noted that strictly speaking 'preformation' theory held that the formation of each new being took place through the activities of the soul or spirit in the parents' body whereas only 'pre-existence' theory or 'emboîtement' held that all organisms were created at one time in the past. See Peter Bowler, 'Preformation and pre-existence in the seventeenth century', *Journal of the History of Biology*, 4 (1971), 221–44.

[50] George Garden, 'A discourse concerning the modern theory of generation', *Philosophical Transactions of the Royal Society*, 196 (1691), 474–8.

[51] In addition to the ovists and animalculists there was a third and even more bizarre school of thought, that of the 'panspermists' who argued that all beings were created by God at one moment in time, that such tiny beings were suspended in the atmosphere and that they passed from the air into the man and then into the woman and then were born. For example William Wollaston wrote that all souls were created in the beginning but the material form of beings was effected later.

> If then the *semina* out of which animals are produced, are (as I doubt not) *animalcula* already formed; which, being dispersed about, especially in some opportune places, are *taken in* with aliment, or perhaps the very air; being separated in the bodies of the *males* by strainers proper to every kind, and then lodged in *their* seminal vessels, do *there* receive some kind of addition and influence; and being thence transferred into the wombs of the females, are *there* nourished more plentifully, and grow, till they become too big, to be longer confined.

(N.N. [William Wollaston], *The Religion of Nature Delineated* (London,

1722), 65.) Microscopic studies were thus turned to the purposes of Christian apology.

[52] Swammerdam cited in Adelman, *Malpighi*, II, 908.

[53] John Wilkins, *Of the Principles and Duties of Natural Religion* (London, 1673), 83; William Paley, *Natural Theology* (London: Fauldner, 1802), and see also John Ray, *The Wisdom of God Manifested in the Works of Generation* (London: Smith, 1691).

[54] Michael H. Hoffheimer, 'Maupertuis and the eighteenth-century critique of pre-existence', *Journal of the History of Biology*, 15 (1982), 119–44.

[55] Louis A. Landa, 'The Shandean Homunculus: The background of Sterne's "Little Gentleman"', in Carol Camden (ed.), *Restoration and Eighteenth Century Literature* (Chicago: University of Chicago Press, 1963), 49–68.

[56] W. Smellie, *A Treatise on the Theory and Practice of Midwifery* (London: Wilson, 1752), 115; see also Hamilton, *Midwifery*, 40.

[57] On doctors' appreciation of the embryological debate at the end of the eighteenth century see for example John Aitken, *Principles of Midwifery* (Edinburgh: 1785), 42–4 and Charles Severn, *First Lines on the Practice of Midwifery* (London: S. Highley, 1831), 31. On the scientific level see Shirley A. Roe, *Matter, Life and Generation: Eighteenth-century embryology and the Haller-Wolff debate* (Cambridge: Cambridge University Press, 1981).

[58] See for example Roger's work cited in note 42.

[59] Hilda Smith anachronistically attacks seventeenth-century writers such as Culpeper for not adopting a 'straightforward informational approach' in their discussion of gynaecology and so implies that in a scientifically based medicine social and sexual preoccupations would not intrude. This chapter argues that such an overlap always occurs. See Hilda Smith, 'Gynecology and ideology in seventeenth-century England', in Berenice A. Caroll (ed.), *Liberating Women's History* (Urbana: University of Illinois Press, 1976), 97–115.

[60] Harvey, *Works*, 298–9.

[61] M. de la Vauguion, *A Compleat Body of Chirurgical Operations* (1699), cited in Eccles, *Obstetrics*, 35.

[62] Procope-Couteau, *L'Art*, 25.

[63] A Physician, *Speculations on the Mode and Appearances of Impregnation in the Human Female* (Edinburgh, n.p., 1789), 43.

[64] F. E. Fodéré cited in Michael Ryan, *The Philosophy of Marriage* (London, n.p., 1837), 331.

[65] Dr William Acton, *The Functions and Disorders of the Reproductive Organs* (London: J. A. Churchill, 1857), 213 and see also John S. and Robin M. Haller, *The Physician and Sexuality in Victorian America* (Urbana: University of Illinois Press, 1974), 96–101.

[66] James Marion Sims, *Clinical Notes on Uterine Surgery* (London: n.p. 1866), 369.

[67] E. H. East, *A Treatise of the Pleas of the Crown* (London, 1803), I, 445, and see also Susan S. M. Edwards, *Female Sexuality and the Law* (Oxford: Martin Robertson, 1981), 123–4.

[68] M. Quinland, *Victorian Prelude* (New York: Archon, 1941); Peter Fryer, *Mrs. Grundy: Studies in English Prudery* (London: Maxwell, 1963).

[69] Stephen Nissenbaum, *Sex, Diet, and Debility in Jacksonian America: Sylvester Graham and Health Reform* (Westport, Conn.: Greenwood, 1980), 28; Charles E. Rosenberg, 'Sexuality, class, and race in nineteenth-century America', *American Quarterly*, 25 (1973), 131–53.

[70] Peter Cominos, 'Innocent femina sensualis in unconscious conflict', in Martha Vicinus (ed.), *Suffer and Be Still: Women in the Victorian age* (Bloomington: University of Indiana Press, 1972; London: Methuen, 1980), 158–62.

[71] Nancy F. Cott, 'Passionlessness: an interpretation of Victorian sexual ideology, 1790–1850', *Signs*, 4 (1978), 219–36.

[72] Carolyn Merchant has some interesting things to say about the rise of the 'machine metaphor' in late seventeenth-century medical discussions of women's sexual passivity, but in presenting male chauvinism as unchanging from Aristotle to Harvey to Darwin she fails to produce a believable explanation of shifts in attitudes towards procreation. See *The Death of Nature: Women, ecology, and the scientific movement* (San Francisco: Harper-Row, 1980).

[73] Margaret Jacob, *The Newtonians and the English Revolution, 1689–1720* (Ithaca: Cornell University Press, 1976) and on eighteenth-century enlightenment, thought and women see also Jacob's *The Radical Enlightenment: Pantheists, freemasons, and republicans* (London: Allen & Unwin, 1981), 208.

[74] Marlene Legates, 'The cult of womanhood in eighteenth-century thought', *Eighteenth Century Studies*, 10 (1976), 21–40; A. D. Harvey, '*Clarissa* and the Puritan tradition', *Essays in Criticism*, 28 (1978), 38–51.

[75] Carl Degler has attacked the notion that Victorian doctors denied women's sexuality and has asserted that 'it was recognized that the sex drive was so strong in a woman that to deny it might well compromise her health'. But to make his case Degler has to rely on works written in the 1870s and later; the early nineteenth-century material which would undermine his argument is ignored. See Carl N. Degler, 'What ought to be and what was: women's sexuality in the nineteenth century', *American Historical Review*, 79 (1974), 1467–90; *At Odds: Women and the family in America from the Revolution to the present* (New York: Oxford University Press, 1980). That sexual repression percolated down to the working classes is indicated by the inability of nineteenth-century artisan autobiographers to discuss their sex lives. See David Vincent, 'Love and death and the nineteenth-century working class', *Social History*, 5 (1980), 223–48.

2 'To remedy barrenness and to promote the faculty of generation'

[1] Thomas Cogan, *The Haven of Health* (London: Henric Midleton, 1584), 240, cited in Lawrence Babb, 'The physiological conception of love in the Elizabethan and early Stuart drama', *Proceedings of the Modern Language Association* (1941), 1020.

[2] See, for example, Cogan, *The Haven of Health*, 241–7; Francis Bacon, *History Natural and Experimental of Life and Death* (London: W. Lee, 1638).

[3] Robert Burton, *The Anatomy of Melancholy* (London: Bell, 1896, first edn 1621), III, 66.

[4] John Archer (chymical physician), *Every Man His Own Doctor* (London: Peter Lillicrap, 1671), 103.

[5] Levine Lemnie, *The Touchstone of Complexions*, tr. T. Newton (London: Barth, 1581), 43; Thomas Newton, *An Herbal* (London: Bellifont, 1587).

[6] Sir Thomas Browne, *Common Errors* in S. Wilkin (ed.), *Sir Thomas Browne's Works* (London: Pickering, 1835) III, 316; Philip Barrough, *The Method of Physicke* (London: Vautroullier, 1583), 142. See also Dr Christopher Wirtzung, *Praxis: Medicinae universalis: or a General Practice of Physicke* (London: Bishop, 1598), 294–6; Thomas Elyot, *Castel of Health* (London, 1541), 27; John Jones, *A Brief, Excellent and Profitable Discourse, of the Natural Beginning of all Growing and Living Things* (London: L. Jones, 1574); N. Culpeper, *Galen's Art of Physick* (London: Cole, 1652).

[7] William Coles, *The Art of Simpling* (London: Brook, 1656), 3 and the same author's *Adam in Eden, or Nature's Paradise* (London: John Streater, 1657). On the doctrine of signatures see also Oswald Crollius, *Traicté des signatures* (Paris, 1633), Jollivet Castelot, *La médecine spagyrique* (Paris: Durville, 1912), and Jacob Boehme, *Signatura Rerum: The Signature of All Things* (New York: Everyman, 1934).

[8] Coles, *Adam*, 628.

[9] *Romeo and Juliet*, II, 3.

[10] John Ray, *A Collection of English Proverbs* (Cambridge: Hayes, 1678), 56.

[11] [Rembert Dodoens], *Ram's Little Dodeon* [sic], *A Brief Epitome of a New Herbal* (London: Stafford, 1606); R.C., J.D., M.S., T.B.W.C.M.H., *The Compleat Midwife's Practice Enlarged* (London: N. Brook, 1663), 309; Richard L. Greaves, *Society and Religion in Elizabethan England* (Minneapolis: University of Minnesota Press, 1981), 240.

[12] And see also Francisco Guerra, 'Sex and drugs in the sixteenth century', *British Journal of Addiction*, 18 (1974), 273–87.

[13] Geoffrey Chaucer, *Canterbury Tales* (New York: Bobbs-Merrill, 1971; London: Macmillan 1974), lines 1807–8; see also Sir Kenelm Digby, *Choice and Experimental Receipts in Physick and Chirgery* (London: H. Brome, 1668), 239–40.

[14] Alexander Pope, 'January and May', in G. Tillotson (ed.), *The Poems of Alexander Pope* (London: Methuen, 1940), II, 32–3.

[15] Thomas Otway, *The Soldier's Fortune* in J. C. Ghosh (ed.), *The Works of Thomas Otway* (Oxford: Clarendon, 1932), V.

[16] *The Merry Wives of Windsor*, V, v, 23.

[17] John Dryden, *The Satires of Decimus Junius Juvenalis* (London: Tonson, 1735).

[18] William Langham, *The Garden of Health* (London, 1578); Leonard Sowerby, *The Ladies Dispensatory* (London: Ibbotson, 1651); Robert Pemell, *Tractatus . . . A Treatise of the Nature and Quality of Such Simples* (London: Simmons, 1652); William Turner, *The First and Second Parts of the Herbal of William Turner* (London: Birckman, 1568), II, 70; John Maplet, *A Greene Forest of a Natural Historie* (London: H. Denham, 1567), 38; *An Herbal [Banckes Herbal]* (New York: Scholars Press, 1941), 17; Lemnie, *Complexions*, 81. Even at the end of the eighteenth century an eminent physician like Thomas Percival could write: 'A physician of the first rank in his profession, has suggested to me, that tea may be considered as a powerful aphrodisiac; and he imputes the amazing population of China, amongst other causes, to the general use of it'. See Thomas Percival, *Observations on the State of Population in Manchester* (Manchester: n.p., 1790), 43. Ointments to increase heat and ensure the erection of the male member were also mentioned in some of the medical texts. William Sermon recommended musk and ambergris in *The Ladies Companion, or the English Midwife* (London: Edward Thomas, 1671), 12.

[19] *Othello*, I, ii.

[20] John Aubrey, *Remaines of Gentilisme and Judaisme* (1686–87), in *Three Prose Works* (Carbondale: Southern Illinois University Press, 1972), 351.

[21] Francis Beaumont and John Fletcher, *Philastre* (1610), in *Works* (Cambridge: Cambridge University Press, 1910), IV, i; John Gay, *The Shepherd's Week* (1714) (London: Scolar Press, 1969), 38.

[22] See for example, *Aristotle's Compleat Masterpiece* (London: Booksellers, 1727?), 55.

[23] Elizabeth Okeover, 'Collection of Receipts', c. 1700, Wellcome MS 3712; Grace Springatt, 'Receipt Book', c. 1686, Wellcome MS 4683; Rebecca Tallany, 'Her Booke', c. 1736, Wellcome MS 4572. See also Hannah Woolley, *The Accomplish'd Lady's Delight* (London: Harris, 1672), 132; Elizabeth Smith, *The Compleat Housewife* (London, 1725), 249; A Physician, *The Ladies Physical Directory* (London, n.p., 1727); John Ball, *The Female Physician* (London: Davis, 1770), 70; Bath and Tunbridge Wells would owe much of their early eighteenth-century popularity to the supposedly fecundicating powers of their waters. See R. S. Neale, *Bath, 1680–1850: A Social History* (London: Routledge & Kegan Paul, 1981), 15. The developers of spas and writers of medical manuals thus exploited in a new way the old fear of barrenness. See for

example Matthew Mackaile, *Moffet-Well or, A Topographico-Spagyricall Description of the Mineral Wells* (Edinburgh: Brown, 1664).

[24] Nicholas Culpeper, *A Directory for Midwives* (London: Cole, 1656), 97. See also William Sermon, *The Ladies Companion or English Midwife* (London: Thomas, 1671), 16.

[25] Katherine Boyle, 'Receipt Book', c. 1634–91, Wellcome MS 1340. Compare to the idea that the woman who uses a prostitute's mirror becomes wanton in C. G. Navert, *Agrippa and the Crisis of Renaissance Thought* (Urbana: University of Illinois Press, 1965), 268.

[26] Cited in Herbert Thomas, *Chapters in American Obstetrics* (Springfield, Illinois: Thomas, 1933), 4. See also Genesis, xxx, 14; Boorde, *Dyetary*, xx, 281; William Westmacott, *A Scripture Herbal* (London: Salisbury, 1694), 107; Browne, *Common Errors*, III, 312–16; Mrs Gutch and Mabel Peacock, *Examples of Printed Folklore, Concerning Lincolnshire* (London: Nutt, 1908), 118.

[27] The World Health Organisation has identified three to four thousand plants used as fertility-regulating agents; their analysis has only just begun. See R. N. Shain and C. J. Paverstein, *Fertility Control* (New York: Harper & Row, 1980), 248.

[28] See Keith Thomas, *Religion and the Decline of Magic: Studies in popular beliefs in sixteenth- and seventeenth-century England* (Harmondsworth: Penguin, 1971), 213; John Baptista Porta, *Natural Magick* (London: Young, 1658).

[29] Lazarus Riverius, *The Practice of Physick* (London: Cole, 1658), 504–5.

[30] Revd Montagu Summers (ed.), *Malleus Maleficarum* (New York: Blom, 1928), 167; see also E. Le Roy Ladurie, *The Mind and the Method of the Historian* (Chicago: University of Chicago Press, 1981), 88.

[31] John Dryden et al., *Ovid's Episteles, with his Amours* (London: J. Tonson, 1729), 323.

[32] Cited in G. L. Kittredge, *Witchcraft in Old and New England* (Cambridge, Mass.: Harvard University Press, 1929), 115.

[33] Thomas Dekker, *The Shoemaker's Holiday* (1599), ed. R. L. Smallwood and S. Weeks (Manchester: Manchester University Press, 1979), xii, 65–7.

[34] Thomas Newton, *Tryall of a Man's Owne Selfe* (London, n.p., 1602), 116.

[35] Reginald Scot, *The Discoverie of Witchcraft* (London: W. Brome, 1584), 77; and see also 82. Henry VIII, tiring of Ann Boleyn, asserted that he 'made this marriage seduced by witchcraft; and that this was evident because God did not permit them to have any male issue'. Cited in Summers, *Malleus*, xxi.

[36] A. L. Rowse, *The Case Books of Simon Forman: Sex and society in Shakespeare's age* (London: Weidenfeld & Nicolson, 1974), 84.

[37] Le Roy Ladurie, *Mind*, 88–96; and see also Jean Delumeau, *Catholicism Between Luther and Voltaire: A New View of the Counter-*

Reformation (London: Burnes & Oates, 1977), 161–4.

[38] Jean Bodin, *Démonomanie des sorciers* (Paris: Jean Dupuis, 1580) and see also Henry Bouget, *An Examination of Witches* (1590), ed. M. Summers (London: Rodher, 1929), 91.

[39] Cited in Audrey Eccles, *Obstetrics and Gynaecology in Tudor and Stuart England* (London: Croom Helm, 1982), ch. 8; and see also Ambroise Paré, *On Monsters and Marvels*, tr. Janis L. Pallister (Chicago: University of Chicago Press, 1982), 105–6.

[40] Francis Bacon, *Sylvia Sylvarum* in *Works* (Cambridge: Riverside Press, 1863), V, 110. In Robert Cotgrave, *A Dictionarie of the French and English Tongues* (London: Adam Islip, 1611) 'esguillette nouée' was explained as 'The charming of a man's codpeece point so, as he shall not be able to use his owne wife, or woman (though he may use any other;) Hence; avoir l'esguillette nouée, signifies, to want erection: (This impotence is supposed to come by the force of certaine words uttered by the charmer while he ties a knot on the parties codpeece-point).'

[41] Burton, *Melancholy*, 288.

[42] Thomas Heywood and Richard Brome, *The Late Lancashire Witches* (London: Harper, 1634), IV, 3 (H3). Brian Easlea notes another satire on the same theme:

> In 'The [London] Women's Petition against Coffee' the introduction of Turkish coffee was identified as the cause of what was claimed to be London men's sexual shortcomings. According to the petition the continual sipping of this 'little, *base, black, thick, nasty, bitter, nauseous* Puddle water' was alone sufficient to tie up 'the *Codpiece-point*' – witches' charms being no longer necessary! – as proved by the fact that 'this ugly *Turkish* Enchantress' had already grievously 'Eunucht our Husbands and *Crippled* our more kind *gallants*, that they are become as Impotent as Age'.

Science and Sexual Oppression: Patriarchy's confrontation with women and nature (London: Weidenfeld & Nicolson, 1981), 78.

[43] Culpeper, *Directory*, 89.

[44] Jane Sharp, *The Compleat Midwife's Companion: or the Art of Midwifery Improved* (London: Marshall, 1725), 69; and see also Daniel Defoe, *Conjugal Lewdness* (London: Warner, 1727), 163.

[45] R.C., *Compleat Midwife*, 220. It is obvious enough why the stallion or stonehorse would have purportedly magical, virile qualities; so too did a herb called stonehorse or English Prick-my-dame or Prick-madam.

[46] John Webster, *The Displaying of Supposed Witchcraft* (London: S.M., 1677), 246.

[47] Bacon, *Sylvia*, V, 110.

[48] R. N. Shain and C. J. Paverstein, *Fertility Control* (New York: Harper & Row), 248.

[49] Bacon, *Sylvia*, V, 146.

[50] J. G. Frazer, *The Golden Bough: A study in magic and religion* (London: 1922; new edn Macmillan 1963), 314–17. In the Scottish ballad 'Willie's Ladie' a woman prevents the birth of her grandchild with 'nine witch knots'. See F. J. Child, *The English and Scottish Popular Ballads* (New York: Folklore Press, 1957), I, 81–8. The last witchcraft trial in Ireland which took place in 1711 also involved knots. See St John D. Seymour, *Irish Witchcraft and Demonology* (Dublin: Hodge, Figgis, 1913), 208; *Folklore*, 33 (1922), 291–2.

[51] See Pemell, *Tractatus*, 157; Browne, *Common Errors*, III, 178; and E. A. Wallis Budge, *Amulets and Superstitions* (Oxford: Oxford University Press, 1930), 308–17.

[52] Thomas, *Religion*, 222.

[53] Lemnie, *Touchstone*, 270; Bacon, *Sylvia*, #154; and see also Louise Bourgeois, *Observations diverses sur la stérilité* (Paris: Dehours, 1617), 27; John Brand, *Observations on the Popular Antiquities of Great Britain* (1795) (New York: AMS Press, 1970), III, 282.

[54] Coles, *Simpling*, 71; see also T. Lupton, *A Thousand Notable Things* (London: Wilkie, 1776), 83.

[55] On the use of such charms by the Anglo-Saxons see Dr G. Stone, *Anglo-Saxon Magic* (Hague: Martinus Nijhof, 1948), 196–205; William Bonser, *The Medical Background of Anglo-Saxon England* (London: Wellcome, 1963), 265 ff.: and see also Revd Thomas Oswald Cockayne, *Leechdome, Wortcunning, and Starcraft of Early Modern England*, ed. C. Singer (London: Holland Press, 1961, first edn 1864–1866), 3 vols.

[56] Dr Jacques Ferrand, *Love Melancholy* (Oxford, 1640), 310.

[57] Gaule cited in Brand, *Antiquities*, II, 325.

[58] Henry Bourne, *Antiquates Vulgares; or the Antiquities of the Common People* (1725) cited in Brand, *Antiquities*, II, 325.

[59] *Aristotle's Masterpiece: or the Secrets of Generation* (London: W.B., 1690), 80.

[60] As proof Walter Charlton notes, 'It hath been observed, that in men excessively addicted to women, the Brain it self is not only much debilitated, but made also lax, thin, and watery'. *Natural History of Nutrition, Life, and Voluntary Motion* (London: Henry Hetherington, 1659), 161; see also Burton, *Melancholy*, III, 223.

[61] Barrough, *Physick*, 157.

[62] Timothy Bright, *A Treatise on Melancholie* (1586) (New York: Da Capo Press, 1969), 176.

[63] Burton, *Melancholy*, III, 67. See also Rabelais, *Gargantua and Pantagruel* (London: Bibliophilist Society, n.d.), 324–5.

[64] J. Huarte Navarro, *The Examination of Men's Wits* (London: Adam Fillip, 1594), 292.

[65] Anon., *The Family Companion for Health* (London: Fayram, 1729), 5. For similar reasons in the sixteenth century it was asserted that dancers did not menstruate. See Barrough, *Physick*, 145.

166

[66] Percival, *Observations*, 44.

[67] Nicolas Venette, *Conjugal Love Reveal'd* (London: Hinton, 1720), 125.

[68] Venette, *Conjugal Love*, 128.

[69] *Aristotle's Masterpiece* (1690), 174.

[70] Plato cited in Daniel Rogers, *Matrimonial Honour* (London: Harper, 1642), 178; A. F. M. Willich, *Lectures on Diet and Regimen* (London: Longman, 1799), 501.

[71] Burton, *Melancholy*, III, 317.

[72] R. Bunworth, *The Doctoresse* (London: Bourne, 1656), 50.

[73] Nicolas Fontanus, *The Womans Doctor* (London: Howes, 1652), 137.

[74] Bernard Capp, *Astrology and the Popular Press, 1500–1800* (London: Faber & Faber, 1979), 120; and see also Pierre de Brantôme, *Love of Fair and Gallant Ladies* (1560) (London: Fortune Press, n.d.), 122–4.

[75] Sharp, *Midwife*, 70.

[76] Sermon, *Ladies Companion*, 18.

[77] Owen Wood, *An Alphabetical Book of Physical Secrets* (London: John Norton, 1639), 233; and see also I. Fletcher, *The Differences, Causes, and Judgements of Urine* (London: John Legatt, 1641), 73–7.

[78] Boyle, MS 1340. See also *Aristotle's Masterpiece* (1690), 114.

[79] John Cotta, *Short Discoverie* (London: Jones, 1612); Thomas Ross (ed.), *A Book of Elizabethan Magic: Thomas Hill's natural and artificial conclusions* (1567) (Regensburg: Verlag Hans Carl, 1974), 68; Lucille B. Pinto, 'The folk practice of gynecology and obstetrics in the Middle Ages', *Bulletin of the History of Medicine*, 47 (1973), 513–23. For an attack on the belief in the ability to detect pregnancy and sex of child see James Primerose, *Popular Errours, or the Errours of the People in Physick*, tr. Robert Wittie (London: W. Wilson, 1651), 64, 74.

[80] James Guillemeau, *Child-Birth or, the Happy Deliverie of Women* (London: Hatfield, 1612), 8; and see also R.C., *Compleat Midwife*, 73; Culpeper, *Directory*, 103.

[81] Lawrence Stone, *The Crisis of the Aristocracy, 1558–1641* (Oxford: Clarendon, 1965), 589. For a personal account of the risks run see *The Autobiography of Mrs Alice Thornton* (London: Quaritch, 1875), Surtees Society, vol. 62. On spontaneous abortion in the twentieth century see Edward Shorter, *A History of Women's Bodies* (New York: Basic Books, 1982), 193.

[82] Queen Elizabeth in *King Henry VI*, Part III, avoids the passions to protect her pregnancy:

And I the rather wean me from despair
For love of Edward's offspring in my womb
This is it that makes me bridle passion
And bear with mildness my misfortunes cross,
Ay, ay, for this I draw in many a tear

And stop the rising of blood-sucking sighs,
Lest with my sighs or tears I blast or drown
King Edward's fruit, true heir to th'English crown.

(IV, iv, 17–24)

See also Anon., *Family Companion*, 167; William Salmon, *The Family Dictionary* (London: Rhodes, 1705), 188; Thomas Beddoes, *Hygeia* (Bristol: Mills, 1803), I, 82; A. Hume, *Every Woman Her Own Physician or, the Lady's Medical Assistant* (London: Richardson & Urquhart, 1776), 86.

[83] Sermon, *Ladies Companion*, 23.

[84] Walter Harris, *An Exact Enquiry Into, and Care of the Acute Diseases of Infants* (London: Clement, 1693), 13. See also Venette, *Conjugal Love*, 121.

[85] John Pechey, *The Complete Midwife's Practice Enlarged* (London: Rhodes, 1698), 65. See also Sermon, *Ladies Companion*, 41.

[86] Ann Brumwich, 'Her Booke', c. 1650, Wellcome MS 160; Tallany, Wellcome MS 4572.

[87] Anonymous seventeenth-century Wellcome MS 635; Hannah Woolley, *The Gentlewoman's Companion or, A Guide to the Female Sex* (London: Maxwell, 1675), 181.

[88] Robert Pemell, *The Second Part of the Treatise . . . of Physical Simples* (London: Legatt, 1653); Anon., *The Compleat Herbal or, Family Physician* (Manchester: Swindall, 1787), II, 147; and see also Michael K. Eshleman, 'Diet during pregnancy in the sixteenth and seventeenth centuries', *Journal of the History of Medicine and Allied Sciences*, 30 (1975), 23–39.

[89] Johanna St John, 'Her Booke', c. 1680, Wellcome MS 4338.

[90] T. J. Pettigrew, *On Superstitions Connected with Medicine and Surgery* (London: John Churchill, 1844), 85; Browne, *Common Errors*, II, 305.

[91] Walter Harris, *Pharmacologia Anti-Empirica, or a Rationale Discourse of Remedies* (London: Chiswell, 1683), 312.

[92] William Salmon, *Collecteana Medica: The Country Physician* (London: Taylor, 1703), 55, 299–300; see also Brand, *Antiquities*, II, 67.

[93] Ann Brumwich, 'Her Booke', c. 1650, Wellcome MS 160, 215; John Hall, *Select Observations on English Bodies* (London: Shirley, 1679), 49 and see also Hannah Woolley, *The Accomplish'd Lady's Delight* (London: Harris, 1677), 125.

[94] See W. G. Black, *Folk Medicine* (London: Folklore Society, 1883), 84, 90 and Beryl Rowland, *Medieval Woman's Guide to Health: The First English Gynaecological Handbook* (London: Croom Helm, 1981), 32–3.

[95] John Bale, *Comedye Concernynge Thre Lawes, Moses and Christ* (1538) (New York, AMS Press, 1970), E III.

[96] Bale, *Comedye*, B III.

[97] Brand, *Antiquities*, II, 68.

[98] Pettigrew, *Superstitions*, 85; Brand, *Antiquities*, II, 69.

99 Cited in William Jones, *Credulities Past and Present* (London: Chatto & Windus, 1880), 388. See also T. R. Forbes, *The Midwife and the Witch* (New Haven: Yale University Press, 1966), 67–8.

100 See Paul Slack, 'Mirrors of health and treatises of poor men: the uses of the vernacular medical literature of Tudor England', in Charles Webster (ed.), *Health, Medicine and Mortality in the Seventeenth Century* (Cambridge: Cambridge University Press, 1979), 237–73.

101 Harris, *Enquiry*, II; see also Nathaniel Highmore, *The History of Generation* (London: John Martin, 1651), 95–6.

102 Bouget, *Witches*, 30 and see also Aubrey, *Works*, 351; Harris, *Enquiry*, 12–14; Browne, *Common Errors*, III, 183. Even a man, overcome by some craving or desire, would in the seventeenth century be said 'to be with child'. Thus Pepys reported in his *Diary*, 14 May 1660, 'I sent my boy, who like myself, is with child to see any strange thing'. F. P. Wilson (ed.), *The Oxford Dictionary of English Proverbs* (Oxford: Clarendon, 1970), 119.

103 G. J. Witkowski, *Histoire des accouchements chez tous les peuples* (Paris: Steinheil, n.d.), 170. For a twentieth-century analysis of pregnant women's 'longings' see Hilary Graham, 'The social image of pregnancy: pregnancy as spirit possession', *Sociological Review*, 24 (1976), 291–308; Ioan Lewis, *Ecstatic Religion: An anthropological study of spirit possession and Shamanism* (Harmondsworth: Penguin, 1971).

104 J. A. Blondel, *The Strength of Imagination in Pregnant Women Examin'd* (London: Peele, 1729). See also Daniel Turner, *The Force of the Mother's Imagination . . . Still Further Considered* (London: Walthoe, 1730) and Katherine Park and Lorraine J. Daston, 'Unnatural conceptions: the study of monsters in sixteenth- and seventeenth-century France and England', *Past and Present*, 92 (1981), 20–54. David Hartley devoted a chapter 'To examine how far the longings of pregnant women are agreeable to the doctrines of vibrations and associations' in *Observations on Man* (London: Richardson, 1749), I, 164–6.

105 *Ram's Little Dodeon*, 138; G.W., *A Rich Storehouse or Treasury for the Diseased* (London: Badger, 1631), 91 ff.; Mrs Neville, 'Receipt Book', c. 1720, Wellcome MS 3685.

106 Jane Baber, 'A Book of Receipts', seventeenth century, Wellcome MS 108; R.C., *Compleat Midwife*, 303; Anon., *The Compleat Servant-Maid or, The Young Maiden's Tutor* (London: Tracy, 1700).

107 Eccles, *Obstetrics*.

108 *The Grete Herbal*, tr. Peter Treveris (London, 1526), cccc; Turner, *Herbal*, and see also Anon., *Compleat Herbal*, 140; E.S., *The Compleat Housewife* (London: J. Pemberton, 1729), 280.

109 *An Herbal* (1525), 43, 49; Rebecca Tallany, 'Her Book of Recipes', Wellcome MS 4572; Lady Sleighs, 'Lady Sleighs Bookes', c. 1647, Wellcome MS 751; Pemell, *Simples*.

110 Philip Barrough, *The Method of Physick* (London: A. Miller, 1652), 203.

111 Letitia Owen, 'Household Book', c. 1720–1749, Wellcome MS

3731; Grace Acton, 'Household Book', eighteenth century, Wellcome MS 1.

[112] Black, *Folk Medicine*, 178.

[113] Kittredge, *Witchcraft*, 115; see also Aubrey, *Works*, 252.

[114] Kittredge, *Witchcraft*, 115.

[115] J. G. Frazer, *The Golden Bough: A study in magic and religion* (London: Macmillan, 1963, first edn 1922), 320. See also I, 70 of the 1911 edition.

[116] Mary Preston, 'Recipe Book', *c.* 1725, Wellcome MS 3087.

[117] Johanna St John, Wellcome MS 4338.

[118] Langham, *Garden*, 547; see also Peter Levens, *A Right Profitable Book for all Diseases* (London: White, 1582), 105–7. On actual delivery processes see Eccles, *Obstetrics* and Nicole Belmont, *Les signes de la naissance* (Paris: Plon, 1971).

[119] Aphra Behn (?), *The Ten Pleasures of Matrimony* (London: Navarre, 1950, 1st edn 1682), 50, 51, 53, 68, 94, 98.

[120] William Cadogan, *An Essay Upon Nursing and the Management of Children* (London: J. Roberts, 1748, 6th edn 1753), 3, 4, 29, and see also John Rendle-Short, 'Infant management in the eighteenth century, with special reference to the work of William Cadogan', *Bulletin of the History of Medicine*, 34 (1960), 97–122.

[121] William Heberden, *An Epitome of Infantile Disorders* (London: Lackington, 1805), xii.

[122] James Nelson, *An Essay on the Government of Children* (London: Dodsley, 1753), 153.

[123] James Makitrick Adair, *Medical Cautions* (London: Dodsley, 1786), 159.

[124] James Parkinson, *Medical Admonitions to Families* (London: Symonds, 1801), 8; and see also James Parkinson, *The Villager's Friend and Physician* (London: Symonds, 1804), 5–6, 66–9. Some doctors acknowledged the fact that midwives were indispensable; the answer was to make sure they were instructed. See Valentine Seaman, *The Midwives Monitor and Mothers Mirror* (New York: Isaac Collins, 1800).

[125] See, for example, Joseph Bingham, *Origines ecclesiasticae or the Antiquities of the Christian Church* (London: Knaplock, 1710–22); M. L. Saucerotte, *Examen de plusiers préjugés et usages abusifs concernant les femmes enceintes* (Strasbourg: Gay, 1777). On the clash between the low and high cultures see Natalie Z. Davis, 'Proverbial wisdom and popular errors', *Society and Culture in Sixteenth-Century France* (Stanford: Stanford University Press, 1975), 227–70; Charles E. Rosenberg, 'The therapeutic revolution: medicine, meaning, and social change in nineteenth-century America', *Perspectives in Biology and Medicine*, 20 (1977), 485–506; Margaret Conner Versluysen, 'Old wives' tales? Women healers in English history', in Colin Davies (ed.), *Rewriting Nursing History* (London: Croom Helm, 1980), 175–200; Richard M. Dorson, *The British Folklorists: A history* (Chicago: University of Chicago Press, 1968), 1–30.

126 John Arbuthnot and Alexander Pope, *Memoirs of the Extraordinary Life, Works, and Discoveries of Martinus Scriblerus*, ed. C. Kerby-Miller (New Haven: Yale University Press, 1950), 96; and see also G. R. Rousseau, 'Pineapples, pregnancy, pica and *Peregrine Pickle*', in G. R. Rousseau and P. G. Boucé, *Tobias Smollett: Bicentennial essays presented to Lewis M. Knapp* (New York: Oxford University Press, 1971), 79–110.

127 Eccles, *Obstetrics*, 121.

128 See Edward Shorter, *A History of Women's Bodies* (New York: Basic Books, 1982), 51–90; on deaths of mothers see B. M. Willmott Dobbie, 'Attempts to estimate the true rate of maternal mortality, sixteenth to eighteenth centuries', *Medical History*, 26 (1982), 79–90.

129 See L. J. Jordanova, 'Natural facts: a historical perspective on science and sexuality', in Carol MacCormack and Marilyn Strathern (eds), *Nature, Culture and Gender* (Cambridge: Cambridge University Press, 1980), 42–69. On the decline of herbal beliefs see Scott Atran, 'Covert fragmenta and the origins of the botanical family', *Man*, 18 (1983), 51–71.

130 Carol P. MacCormack (ed.), *Ethnography of Fertility and Birth* (London: Academic Press, 1982).

131 See for example Christopher Hill, *Economic Problems of the Church* (Oxford: Clarendon, 1956), 168, and Peter Rushton, 'Purification or social control? Ideologies of reproduction and the churching of women after childbirth', BSA Annual Conference paper, Manchester, 1982.

132 Clellan Stearns Ford, *A Comparative Study of Human Reproduction* (New Haven: Yale Publications in Anthropology, no. 32, 1945), 36–9.

3 'Excellent recipes to keep from bearing children'

1 J. Knodel and E. van de Walle, 'Lessons from the past: policy implications of historical fertility studies', *Population and Development Review*, 5 (1979), 227.

2 Orest and Patricia Ranum (eds), *Popular Attitudes Towards Birth Control in Pre-Industrial France and England* (New York: Harper & Row, 1972), 10–20.

3 See Steven Polgar, 'Population history and population policies from an anthropological perspective', *Current Anthropology*, 13 (1972), 203–11.

4 Pierre J. Payer, 'Early medieval regulations concerning marital sexual relations', *Journal of Medieval History* 6 (1980), 353–76; P. P. A. Buller, 'Birth control in the west in the thirteenth and fourteenth centuries', *Past and Present* 94 (1982), 3–26.

5 Jaroslav Pelikan (ed.), *Luther's Works* (St Louis: Concordia, 1965), VII, 21.

6 Christopher Hooke, *The Child-Birth or Woman's Lecture* (London: Orwin, 1590), B5.

7 T. Hilder, *Conjugall Counsell* (London: Stafford, 1653), 18, 21.

[8] Nicholas Culpeper, *A Directory for Midwives* (London: Peter Cole, 1660), 70.

[9] Richard Smalbroke, *Reformation Necessary to Prevent our Ruin* (London: Downing, 1728), 22.

[10] Joyce Oldham Appleby, *Economic Thought and Ideology in Seventeenth-Century England* (Princeton: Princeton University Press, 1978), 135 ff.; R. R. Kuczynski, 'British demographers on fertility, 1660–1760', in Lancelot Hogben, *Political Arithmetic: A Symposium of Population Studies* (London: Allen & Unwin, 1938), 283–330.

[11] Thomas Hobbes, *The Elements of Law* (1640) in *Works*, ed. Sir William Molesworth (London: 1839–45), IV, 214–15.

[12] John Graunt, *Natural and Political Observations . . . Upon the Bills of Mortality* (London: n.p., 1662), and see also John Disney, *An Essay Upon the Execution of the Laws Against Immorality and Prophaneness* (London: Downey, 1720), xiv–xv.

[13] 'Populadia', *A Discourse Concerning the Having Many Children in Which the Prejudices Against a Numerous Offspring are Removed* (London: Rogers, 1695), 3.

[14] *Guardian*, no. 105 (11 July 1713).

[15] See Ruth McClure, *Coram's Children: The London Foundling Hospital in the Eighteenth Century* (New Haven: Yale University Press, 1981).

[16] Anon., *Some Considerations on the Necessity and Usefulness of the Royal Charter Establishing an Hospital for the Maintenance and Education of Exposed and Deserted Children* (London: Meadow, 1740), 4. See also Thomas Short, *New Observations* (London: Longman, 1750), 162.

[17] Isaac Maddox, Bishop of Worcester, *The Wisdom and Duty of Preserving Destitute Children* (London: Woodfall, 1753), 22–3.

[18] Jonas Hanway, *A Candid Historical Account of the Hospital for the Reception of Exposed and Deserted Young Children* (London: Dodsley, 1759), 10–11 and see also *Virtue in a Humble Life* (London: Dodsley, 1774), I, xxi–xxiii; *The Citizen's Monitor* (London: Dodsley, 1780), 158.

[19] Culpeper, *Directory*.

[20] *The Works of Aristotle: His Complete Masterpiece* (London: L. Hawes, 1772), 37.

[21] Author Reid, *The Pleasures of Matrimony* (Glasgow: n.p., n.d.), 16–17. Pornography is surprisingly unhelpful as a source for information on fertility control. See Roger Thompson, *Unfit for Modest Ears* (London: Macmillan, 1979).

[22] Cited in Randolph Trumbach, *The Rise of the Egalitarian Family* (New York: Academic Press, 1978), 172.

[23] M. Gérard-Gailley (ed.), *Mme de Sévigné: Lettres* (Paris: Pléiade, 1953), I, 433, 437. That men and women might have different opinions on fertility control was indicated by inquisitors asserting that God would condemn 'a mother who when her husband, after copulating with her, says, I hope a child will come of it; and she answers, May the child go to the devil!', Revd Montagu Summers (ed.), *Malleus*

Maleficarum (1487) (New York: Blom, 1928), 142.

[24] Charles Sedley, *Bellamira or, The Mistress* in *Works* (London: Briscoe, 1722), II, 132.

[25] Edmund Hyde, Earl of Clarendon, *A Collection of Several Tracts* (London: Woodward, 1727), 314.

[26] Anon., *Populousness with Oeconomy* (London: Buckland, 1769), 31.

[27] William Whately, *A Care-Cloth or the Cumbers and Troubles of a Marriage* (London: T. Man, 1624), 50–3. William Ramsey, *Conjugium Conjurgium or Some Serious Considerations on Marriage* (London: Bancks, 1673), 152. See the response made by 'A Country Gentleman' (Dryden?), *Marriage Asserted: In Answer to a Book Entitled Conjugium Conjurgium* (London: Herringman, 1674).

[28] S. Dugard, *The Marriages of Cousin Germans* (London: Bowman, 1673), 57–8, 60–1. For a discussion of some of the literature suggestive of a negative attitude on the part of society as a whole to large numbers of progeny in early modern England see A. Macfarlane, 'Modes of reproduction', in G. Hawthorn (ed.), *Population and Development* (London: Cass, 1978), 109–18.

[29] Patricia James, *Population Malthus: His life and times* (London: Routledge & Kegan Paul, 1979), 387.

[30] Lawrence Stone, *The Family, Sex and Marriage in England, 1500–1800* (New York: Harper & Row, 1977; Harmondsworth: Penguin, 1979), 63–6.

[31] Tietze cited in Moni Nag, *Factors Affecting Human Fertility in Nonindustrial Societies: A cross cultural study* (Yale University Publications in Anthropology, no. 66, New Haven, 1962), 75.

[32] Stone, *Family*, 63–5. On the effects of secondary sterility arising from the fact that for physiological reasons the earlier a woman starts to produce children the earlier she finishes see J. Knodel, 'Family limitation and the fertility transition: evidence from the age patterns of fertility in Europe and Asia', *Population Studies*, 31 (1977), 219–49; E. A. Wrigley and R. S. Schofield, 'English population history from family reconstitution: summary results 1600–1799', *Population Studies*, 37 (1983), 157–84; Christopher Wilson, 'Marital fertility in pre-industrial England, 1550–1849' (Cambridge University, unpublished PhD, 1982), 38, 71–96.

[33] Peter Laslett, *Family Life and Illicit Love in Earlier Generations* (Cambridge: Cambridge University Press, 1977), 105; G. R. Quaife, *Wanton Wenches and Wayward Wives: Peasants and illicit sex in early seventeenth-century England* (London: Croom Helm, 1979), 77. Dyer discovered very marked correlations of conceptions by week of the year with periods of festivity and leisure in late sixteenth- and early seventeenth-century England. See A. Dyer, 'Seasonality of baptisms: An urban approach', *Local Population Studies*, 27 (1981), 26–34 and also E. A. Wrigley and R. S. Schofield, *The Population History of England: A reconstitution* (Cambridge: Cambridge University Press, 1981), 291–3.

[34] Etienne and Françine van de Walle, 'Allaitement, stérilité et contraception: les opinions jusqu'au XIXe siècle', *Population*, 27 (1972), 685 ff.

[35] John Ray, *A Collection of English Proverbs* (Cambridge: Hayes, 1678), 26.

[36] Dr T. Laycock, 'Influence of lactation in preventing the occurrence of pregnancy', *Dublin Medical Press* (26 October 1842), 263; see also John Robertson, *Essays and Notes on the Physiology and Diseases of Women and on Practical Midwifery* (London, 1851), 189–95; L. Populous, *Dissertation sur l'allaitement* (Paris: Didot jeune, 1815).

[37] Thomas Bull, *Hints to Mothers* (London: Longman, 1857), 49; 'Concluding report of the infant mortality committees', *Transactions of the Obstetrical Society of London*, 12 (1870), 388–403.

[38] Alexander Milne, *The Principles and Practices of Midwifery* (Edinburgh: Livingstone, 1871), 135.

[39] Gervase Babington, *Certaine Plaine, Brief, and Comfortable Notes, upon every Chapter of Genesis* (London: T. Charde, 1596), 161; see also Daniel Rogers, *Matrimonial Honour* (London: Harper, 1642), 279.

[40] 'An eminent physician', *The Nurses Guide: or, the right method of bringing up young children to which is added an essay on preserving health and prolonging life* (London: Brotherton, 1729), 23.

[41] William Cadogan, *An Essay Upon Nursing and the Management of Children* (London: J. Roberts, 1748); John Nelson, *An Essay on the Governing of Children* (London: Dodsley, 1753); George Armstrong, *An Essay on the Diseases Most Fatal to Infants* (London: T. Cadell, 1771); Michael Underwood, *A Treatise on the Disorders of Childhood* (London: Mathews, 1797), 3 vols.

[42] Luigi Tansillo, *The Nurse*, tr. William Roscoe (Liverpool: J. McCreery, 1798), 11.

[43] W. de Archenholtz, *A Picture of England* (London: Booksellers, 1797), 327.

[44] John Jones, *The Art and Science of Preserving Bodie and Soule* (London: Bynneman, 1579), 14; on Galen see *Works*, R. Green (ed.) (1951), 29.

[45] William Gouge, *Of Domesticall Duties* (London: John Beale, 1626), 131.

[46] 'A.M.', *A Rich Closet of Physical Secrets* (London: Dawson, 1652).

[47] On the post-partum taboo see A. M. Carr-Saunders, *The Population Problem* (Oxford: Oxford University Press, 1922), 175–6; J. F. Saucier, 'Correlates of the long post partum taboo', *Current Anthropology*, 13 (1972), 238–49. Peter Anderson, 'The reproductive role of the human breast', *Current Anthropology*, 24 (1983), 25–45.

[48] Edmund Hyde, Earl of Clarendon, *A Collection of Several Tracts* (London: Woodward, 1727), 314. For a feminist defence of nursing see 'Sophia' (Lady Mary Wortley Montagu?), *Women Not Inferior to Men* (London: Hawkins, 1739), 12.

[49] Randolph Trumbach, *The Rise of the Egalitarian Family: Aristo-cratic kinship and domestic relations in eighteenth-century England* (New York: Academic Press, 1978), 220. In twentieth-century Nigeria the length of the period of abstinence while the mother nurses her baby is also related to the sex of the child.

> From Lafiaga (Kwara State) . . . it was reported that a woman should resume sex relations 36 weeks after delivering a boy but 30 after a girl. Because there is a preference for male offspring, the distinction between abstention periods following the birth of a girl and a boy clearly shows that besides health motivations (impairment to the child at the breast if another is born, and probably for the safety of the woman) the reason for abstinence, at least partly, is family planning.

Gyorgy T. Acsadi, 'Traditional birth control methods in Yorubaland', in J. F. Marshall and S. Polgar (eds), *Culture, Natality, and Family Planning* (Chapel Hill: University of North Carolina Press, 1976), 139.

In addition to the sex of the child the class of the parents could affect nursing patterns. Much of our evidence is specific to higher-status groups. Inhabitants of the wealthier London parishes are known to have used wet nurses in parishes some distance from the city and to have displayed very short birth intervals. Some evidence suggests that these same groups may have changed their behaviour patterns away from very early weaning in the course of the eighteenth century. See V. Fildes, 'Neonatal feeding practices and infant mortality during the eighteenth century', *Journal of Biosocial Science*, 12 (1980), 313–24; R. Finlay, *Population and Metropolis: The demography of London, 1580–1650* (Cambridge: Cambridge University Press, 1981), 94, 146–8.

[50] On attempts to plot the effectiveness of extended nursings as a contraceptive strategy see Dorothy McLaren, 'Fertility, infant mortality, and breast feeding in the eighteenth century', *Medical History*, 22 (1978), 378–96 and 'Nature's contraceptive: wet-nursing and prolonged lactation: the case of Chesham, Buckinghamshire, 1578–1601', *Medical History*, 23 (1979), 421–41. On the demographic impact of breastfeeding in Britain as compared to the continent see E. A. Wrigley and R. Schofield, 'English population history from family reconstitution: summary results 1600–1799', *Population Studies*, 37 (1983), 157–84; Wilson, 'Marital fertility', 135–54; J. Knodel and C. Wilson, 'The secular increase in fecundity in German village populations: an analysis of reproductive histories of couples married 1750–1899', *Population Studies*, 35 (1981), 53–84.

[51] John Burton, *An Essay Towards a Complete New System of Midwifery* (London: Hodges, 1751), 283.

[52] A slightly later schedule was suggested by Navarro who stated that 'a man should meddle with his wife in the carnal act' no later than six or seven days before the period so that the seed could be well rooted

before the flux appeared. See J. Huarte Navarro, *The Examination of Man's Wits*, tr. R. C. Esquire (London: Adam Filip, 1594), 296.

[53] John Sadler, *The Sick Woman's Private Looking Glass* (Norwood, N.J.: W. J. Johnson, 1977 first edn 1656), 120.

[54] John Pechey, *The Compleat Midwife's Practice Enlarged* (London: Rhodes, 1698), 314 ff.; Nicholas Culpeper, *A Directory for Midwives* (London: Cole, 1656), 97.

[55] A. F. M. Willich, *Lectures on Diet and Regimen* (London: Longman, 1799), 501.

[56] John Powers, *Essays on the Female Economy* (London, 1821), 14–28; James Blondel, *Observations on Some of the More Important Diseases of Women* (London: Cox, 1837); Thomas Laycock, *A Treatise on the Nervous Diseases of Women* (London: Longman, 1840), 42–3; S. Mason, *The Philosophy of Female Health* (London: H. Hughes, 1845); Henry Oldham, 'Clinical lecture on the induction of abortion in a case of contracted vagina from cicatrization', *London Medical Gazette*, 9 (1849), 45–8; E. J. Tilt, *On the Preservation of the Health of Women at the Critical Periods of Life* (London: Churchill, 1851).

[57] Laurence Vaux, *A Plaine and Familiar Exposition of the Ten Commandments* (London: Field, 1618), 296.

[58] W. Perkins, *A Golden Chaine: or, the Description of Theologie* (London: J. Legat, 1600), 84; Gouge, *Domesticall Duties*, 130–1. On the 'dangers' of menstrual blood see Patricia Crawford, 'Attitudes towards menstruation in seventeenth-century England', *Past and Present*, 91 (1981), 47–73.

[59] *William Petty Papers* (London: Constable, 1927), I, 156.

[60] 'Is it not you who used to warn us to watch as much as we could the time after purification of the menses when a woman is likely to conceive, and at that time refrain from intercourse, lest a soul be implicated in the flesh? From this it follows that you consider marriage is not to procreate children, but to satiate lust.' St Augustine, *The Morals of the Manichees*, cited in John Noonan, *Contraception: A history of its treatment by Catholic theologians and canonists* (Cambridge, Mass.: Harvard University Press, 1965), 120.

[61] William Sermon, *The Ladies' Companion, or the English Midwife* (London: Edward Thomas, 1671), 15.

[62] H. H. Ploss and P. Bartels, *Woman: A historical, gynaecological and anthropological compendium*, ed. J. Dingwall (London: Heinemann, 1935), II, 290–1.

[63] Norman E. Himes, *Medical History of Contraception* (Baltimore: Williams and Wilkins, 1936), 170–83.

[64] E. Le Roy Ladurie, *Montaillou* (New York: Pantheon, 1980; Harmondsworth: Penguin, 1980).

[65] *Les admirables secrets d'Albert le Grand* (Cologne, n.p., 1722), 124–7.

[66] William Williams, *Occult Physique* (London: T. Leach, 1660), 135.

[67] Leonard Sowerby, *The Ladies Dispensatory* (London: Ibbotson,

1651), 161. The long life of such beliefs is discussed in Enid M. Porter, 'Some folk beliefs of the Fens', *Folklore*, 69–70 (1958–9), 113–14.

[68] Robert V. Schnucker, 'Elizabethan birth control and Puritan attitudes', *Journal of Interdisciplinary History*, 5 (1975), 655–68.

[69] Langham, *The Garden of Health* (London: T. Harpe, 1633), 584.

[70] *Blagrave's Supplement or Enlargement to Mr Nicholas Culpeper's English Physician* (London: Blagrave, 1677), 157.

[71] Sowerby, *Dispensatory*, 141.

[72] John Archer, *A Compendious Herbal* (London: E.C., 1673), 34, 87.

[73] William Coles, *The Art of Simpling* (London: Brook, 1656), 71.

[74] Langham, *Garden*, 680.

[75] See for example Peter Levens, *A Right Profitable Book for all Diseases* (London: White, 1582), 102; John XXI, *The Treasuri of Helth* (London: Coplande, 1558), xliiii; Thomas Hill, *The Profitable Art of Gardening* (London: Bynneman, 1579), 42, 78; Philip Moore, *The Hope of Health* (London: J. Kingston, 1565), 32.

[76] Joseph Miller, *Botanicum officinale; or, a compendious herbal or, family physician* (Manchester: Swindalls, 1787).

[77] Langham, *Garden*, 680. In the 1578 edition see pages 423, 547, 681.

[78] Philip Barrough, *The Method of Physick* (London: R. Field, 1617), 179.

[79] Robert Lovell, *A Compleat Herball* (Oxford: Davis, 1665); John Gerarde, *The Herbal or General History of Plantes* (London: Norton, 1636), 892; Dr Gesner, *A New Jewel of Health* (London: Baker, 1576), 50; William Coles, *Adam in Eden, or Nature's Paradise* (London: John Streater, 1657).

[80] Gerarde, *Herbal*, 1488.

[81] John Frampton, *Joyful Newes Out of the New-Found Worlde* (London: Allde, 1586), 54.

[82] Lovell, *Compleat Herball*.

[83] Ben Jonson, *Epicoene*, IV, iii in *Works* (Oxford: Oxford University Press, 1954), V, 22.

[84] Daniel Defoe, *A Treatise Concerning the Use and Abuse of the Marriage Bed* (London: Warner, 1727), 144–5.

[85] Nag, *Factors*, 133–4. See also Henry de Lazlo and Paul S. Henshaw, 'Plant materials used by primitive peoples to affect fertility', *Science*, 119 (1954), 626–31.

[86] Cited in Noonan, *Contraception*, 28.

[87] Thomas Wright (ed.), *Three Chapters of Letters Relating to the Suppression of Monasteries* (London: Camden Society, 1843), 97.

[88] Babington, *Comfortable Notes*, 278.

[89] Gouge, *Domesticall Duties*, 130; see also Nicholas Culpeper, *A Directory for Midwives* (London: Cole, 1651), 70.

[90] Cited in Quaife, *Wanton Wenches*, 171–2.

[91] Francis Grose, *A Classical Dictionary of the Vulgar Tongue* (London: S. Hooper, 1785).

[92] James Guillemeau, *Child-Birth or, The Happy Deliverie of Women* (London: Hatfield, 1612).

[93] Pierre de Brantôme, *Lives of Fair and Gallant Ladies* (London: Fortune Press, n.d.), 36; *British Medical Journal* (1868), 128.

[94] W. Brodum, MD, *A Guide to Old Age or a Cure for the Indiscretions of Youth* (London: Myers, 1795) and *To the Nervous, Consumptive and Those of Debilitated Constitutions* (London: Myers, 1797); Samuel Solomon, *A Guide to Health* (West Derby: Speed, 1810); Dr James Graham, *A Lecture on the Generation, Increase and Improvement of the Human Species* (London: Graham, 1783); E. Senate, *The Medical Monitor, Containing Observations on the Effects of Early Dissipation* (London: n.p., n.d.); W. Farrer, *A Short Treatise on Onanism, or the Detestable Vice of Self Pollution* (London: Fletcher, 1767).

[95] *On the Crime of Onan* (London: Curll, 1717), 30. For earlier attacks on the practice in more general studies see Richard Baxter, *A Christian Directory or, Body of Practical Divinity* (London: Neville Simmons, 1678), I, 113; John Norris, *The Theory and Regulation of Love* (London: Manship, 1694).

[96] *Eronia* (London: Crouch, 1724), 21.

[97] *Onania* (London: Crouch, n.d., 4th edn), 66, 83.

[98] *Onania* (London: Crouch, 1723, 7th edn), 99. The shifting of the ends of marriage from procreation to companionship was a product of seventeenth-century Puritan thought. See James T. Johnson, 'English Puritan thought on the ends of marriage', *Church History*, 38 (1969), 429–36; John Halkett, *Milton and the Idea of Matrimony* (New Haven: Yale University Press, 1970).

[99] *Onania* (London: Crouch, 1723, 7th edn), 101. See also *A Supplement to the Onania, or the Heinous Sin of Self-Pollution* (London: n.p., n.d.); 'Philo-Castitatis', *Onania Examin'd and Detected* (London: n.p., n.d.); *Letters of Advice from Two Reverend Divines to a Young Gentleman, about a Weighty Case of Conscience* (London: n.p., 1724).

[100] Otho Beall, 'Aristotle's Masterpiece in America: a landmark in the folklore of medicine', *William and Mary Quarterly*, 20 (1963), 207–22; Janet Blackman, 'Popular theories of generation', in John Woodward and David Richards (eds), *Health Care and Popular Medicine in Nineteenth-Century England* (London: Croom Helm, 1977).

[101] *The Works of Aristotle: His Complete Masterpiece* (London: L. Hawes, 1772), 37.

[102] *Conjugal Love* (London: 1720), 125, 128. Venette was first translated in 1703; he relied heavily on J. B. Sinibaldus, *Geneathropeiae* (Rome: n.p., 1642) which was translated in 1658 as *Rare Verities, or the Cabinet of Venus Unlocked*. See D. F. Foxon, 'Libertine literature in England, 1660–1745', *The Book Collector*, 12 (1963), 26–36.

[103] John Armstrong, *Oeconomy of Love* (London: Cooper, 3rd edn 1739).

[104] See Natalie Z. Davis, *Society and Culture in Early Modern France* (Stanford: Stanford University Press, 1975), 124–51.

[105] Anon., 'Kick him Jenny' (London: 11th edn 1737).

[106] See Jean-Louis Flandrin, *Famille, parenté, maison, sexualité dans l'ancienne societé* (Paris: 1976), 212 ff.

[107] Schnucker, 'Birth control', 655–68.

[108] James Ferrand, *Erotomania* (Oxford: Lichfield, 1640).

[109] Sowerby, *Dispensatory*, 262.

[110] See for example Peter Fryer, *The Birth Controllers* (London: Secker & Warburg, 1965); Angus McLaren, *Birth Control in Nineteenth-Century England* (London: Croom Helm, 1978).

[111] Norman E. Himes, *Medical History of Contraception* (Baltimore: William & Wilkins, 1936), 188–201; E. J. Dingwall, 'Early contraceptive sheaths', *British Medical Journal* (3 January 1953), 40–1.

[112] *A Treatise on All the Degrees and Symptoms of the Venereal Disease in Both Sexes* (London: Crouch, 1708), 63–4. Marten cited, in addition to Fallopio, Hercules Saxonica, *Luis venereoe perfectissimus* (1597). See also Casimir Freschot, *Histoire amoureuse et badine du congrès de la ville d'Utrecht* (Liege: n.p., 1714), 166; on Marten see Ralph Strauss, *The Unspeakable Curll* (New York: n.p., 1927), 26, 206.

[113] J. Spinke, *Venus's Botcher* (London: n.p., 1711), 11.

[114] Joseph Cam, *A Rational and Useful Account of the Venereal Disease* (London: Strahan, 8th edn 1737), 46.

[115] *Tatler*, no. 15 (12–14 May 1709).

[116] Francis Grose, *A Classical Dictionary of the Vulgar Tongue* (London: S. Hooper, 1785); Jean Astruc, *A Treatise*, tr. William Barrowby (London: Richardson, 1737), I, 299. See also Giacomo Casanova, *History of My Life*, tr. W. R. Trask (New York: Harcourt Brace, 1967), IV, 68–9; and E. Lennard Bernstein, 'Who was Condom?', *Human Fertility*, 5 (1940), 172–5, 186.

[117] *A Treatise*, I, 300. For similar warnings see Edme Claude Bourru, *L'art de se traiter soi-meme dans les maladies vénériennes* (Paris: Costard, 1770), 238; James Thorn, *An Attempt to Simplify the Treatment of Sexual Diseases* (London: Highley, 1831), 11.

[118] F. A. Pottle (ed.), *Boswell's London Journal* (London: Heinemann, 1966), 298.

[119] *Syphilis* (London: Walthoe, 1717), 74.

[120] Pottle, *Boswell*, 287.

[121] Pottle, *Boswell*, 287.

[122] F. Grose, *Guide to Health, Beauty, Riches and Honour* (London: Hooper, 1783), 11, 12.

[123] Joseph Gay (J. D. Breval), *The Petticoat* (London: Curll, 1716), 30, 31, 35.

[124] White Kennett, *The Machine or Love's Preservative* (London: n.p., 1724), 2–3.

[125] One of the rare references made in the eighteenth century to the sheath's contraceptive powers was made by Lord Hervey who informed Henry Fox in 1726 that he was sending him 'a dozen preservatives from Claps & impediments to procreation'. Robert Halsbad, *Lord Hervey: Eighteenth-century courtier* (Oxford: Clarendon, 1973), 63. The first extended discussions of the condom as a contraceptive appeared in writings of the early birth controllers: Richard Carlile, *Every Woman's Book: or what is love? Containing most important instructions for the prudent regulation of the principle of love and the number of the family* (London: Carlile, 1826); Robert Dale Owen, *Moral Physiology: or a Brief and Plain Treatise on the Population Question* (New York: Wright, 1830; London: Truelove, 1832); Charles Knowlton, *Fruits of Philosophy or, the Private Companion of Young Married People* (New York: n.p., 1832; London: n.p., 1834).

[126] That family limitation had either come early to certain localities or was being practised by specific groups in England, Europe and colonial North America in the seventeenth and eighteenth centuries is discussed in R. Andorka, 'La prévention des naissances en Hongrie dans la région "Ormansag" depuis la fin du XVIIIe siècle', *Population*, 26 (1971), 63–78; 'Un exemple de faible fécondité légitime dans une région de la Hongrie', *Annales de démographie historique* (1972), 25–53; 'Birth control in the eighteenth and nineteenth centuries in some Hungarian villages', *Local Population Studies*, 22 (1979), 38–43; L. Henry, *Anciennes familles genèvoises: étude démographique: 16e–20e siècles* (Paris: Presses Universitaires de France, 1956); D. Gaunt, 'Family planning and the pre-industrial society: some Swedish evidence', in K. Agren *et al.*, *Aristocrats, Farmers, Proletarians: Essays in Swedish demographic history* (Stockholm: Esselte, 1973), 28–59; E. A. Wrigley, 'Family limitation in pre-industrial England', *Economic History Review*, 19 (1966), 82–109; E. A. Wrigley, 'Marital fertility in seventeenth-century Colyton: a note', *Economic History Review*, 31 (1978), 429–36; D. Scott Smith, 'The demographic history of colonial New England', *Journal of Economic History*, 32 (1972), 165–83.

4   *'All manner of art, to the help of drugs and physicians'*

[1] Mary Beth Norton, *Liberty's Daughters: The Revolutionary experience of American women, 1750–1800* (Boston: Little Brown, 1980), 75.

[2] For later developments see Angus McLaren, 'Women's work and the regulation of family size: the question of abortion in the nineteenth century', *History Workshop*, 4 (1977), 70–82; 'Abortion in England, 1890–1914', *Victorian Studies*, 20 (1977), 379–400.

[3] E. A. Wrigley, *Population and History* (London: Weidenfeld & Nicolson, 1969), 127.

[4] James Rueff, *The Expert Midwife* (London: Alchorn, 1637), 58.

[5] Julia Cherry Spruill, *Women's Life and Work in the Southern Colonies* (New York: Russell & Russell, 1938), 325–6.

[6] G. R. Quaife, *Wanton Wenches and Wayward Wives: Peasants and illicit sex in early seventeenth-century England* (London: Croom Helm, 1979), 118.

[7] Daniel Defoe, *Augusta Triumphans, or the way to make London the most flourishing city in the Universe* (London: Roberts, 1728), 10.

[8] E. Hall (ed.), *Miss Weeton's Journal of a Governess* (London: David & Charles, 1969), I, 60; and on other domestics in similar situations see G. Eland (ed.), *Purefoy Letters, 1735–1753* (London: Sidgwick & Jackson, 1931), 137–8; Margaret Powell, *Below Stairs* (London: Peter Davies, 1968), 95–6; J. A. Perkins, 'Unmarried mothers and the Poor Law in Lindsey, 1800–1850' (unpublished paper, University of New South Wales, 1978), 15.

[9] L. C. Wimberly, *Folklore in English and Scottish Ballads* (New York: Ungar, 1928), 361.

[10] E. K. Wells, *The Ballad Tree* (New York: Ronald Press, 1950), 51.

[11] B. H. Bronson, *The Traditional Tunes of the Child Ballads* (Princeton: Princeton University Press, 1954), I, 328; and see also similar poetical references by Garth:

> frail nymphs, by abortion aim
> To lose a substance, to preserve a name.

Sir Samuel Garth, *The Dispensary* (1699) in Dr Samuel Johnson (ed.), *The Works of the English Poets* (London: Miller, 1800), IX, 436; and by Dryden:

> With cruel Art Corinna would destroy
> The Rip'ning Fruit of our repeated Joy.

John Dryden *et al.*, *Ovid's Epistles, with his Amours* (London: Tonson, 1729), elegy xiii.

[12] Mary Wollstonecraft, *The Wrongs of Woman: or Marie, a Fragment* (London: Johnson, 1798), 92–3. For later novelistic versions of seduced women contemplating abortion see W. Talley, *He, or Man Midwifery* (London: Caudwell, 1865), 12; Henry Butler, *Marriage for the Millions: For the lads and lasses of the working classes* (London: Guest, 1875), 11.

[13] Joanna Southcott, *Letters and Communications . . . Lately Written to Jane Towley* (Stourbridge: Heming, 1804), 55.

[14] Thomas Short, *New Observations* (London, 1750), 74.

[15] Alexander Hamilton, *A Treatise on the Management of Female Complaints* (Edinburgh: Hill, 1792), 231.

[16] Anon., *Thoughts Upon the Means of Alleviating the Miseries Attendant Upon Common Prostitution* (London, n.p., 1799), 6–7.

[17] Martha Mears, *The Pupil of Nature: or candid advice to the Fair Sex* (London: Faulder, 1797), 92–3; and see also Anon., *Advice to Unmarried*

Women: To recover and reclaim the fallen and to prevent the fall of others into the snares and consequences of seduction (London: Rivington, 1791), 17.

[18] *The Autobiography of Mrs Alice Thornton*, The Surtees Society, vol. 62 (London, 1875), 164–5; and see also Daniel Defoe, *Conjugal Lewdness: or matrimonial whoredom. A treatise concerning the use and abuse of the marriage bed* (London: Warner, 1727), 164.

[19] John Pechey, *The Compleat Midwife's Practice Enlarged* (London, Rhodes, 1694), 346.

[20] Cited in Randolph Trumbach, *The Rise of the Egalitarian Family: Aristocratic kinship and domestic relations in eighteenth-century England* (New York: Academic Press, 1978), 172.

[21] Rueff, *Expert Midwife*, 61.

[22] John Dryden, *Juvenal: Satyrs* (London: Tonson, 1693), 195.

[23] Scevole de St Marthe, *Paedotrophia; or the Art of Nursing and Rearing Children*, ed. and tr. H. W. Tytler (London: Nichols, 1797), 104.

[24] John Ferriar, *Medical Histories and Reflections* (London: Cadell & Davies, 1795), 207–8. On the plight of the married poor in France see Olwen Hufton, *The Poor of Eighteenth-Century France* (Oxford: Clarendon, 1974), 331.

[25] Alan Macfarlane, *The Family Life of Ralph Josselin: A seventeenth-century clergyman* (Cambridge: Cambridge University Press, 1970), 199–204.

[26] Alan Macfarlane (ed.), *The Diary of Ralph Josselin, 1616–1683* (Oxford: Oxford University Press, 1976), 484–5.

[27] Nancy Mitford (ed.), *The Ladies of Alderley* (London: Hamish Hamilton, 1938), 141–4.

[28] Although it also comes from a nineteenth-century correspondence it is worth noting the discussion of abortion found in the letters of Hertha Marks and Madame Bodichon. The former wrote to say that she believed an American writer's hostility to abortion unwarranted. 'I am in great doubt on the subject, because she does not prove that it harms anyone particularly, and it does not seem to me a dangerous thing to do.' Bodichon replied: 'I think foeticide is a crime; it is false to say that it does not injure the health of the mother; Dr Blackwell and I have talked of this, and I will tell you her opinion.' (Evelyn Sharp, *Hertha Ayrton, 1854–1923: A Memoir* (London: Edward Arnold, 1926), 45.) Prior to 1803 abortion was not a statutory crime and accordingly one would expect to have found many women of Miss Marks's persuasion.

[29] C. H. L'Estrange Ewen, *Witchcraft and Demonism* (London: Heath Cranton, 1953), 41, 52, 77.

[30] Montagu Summers (ed.), *Malleus Maleficarum* (London: Pushkin Press, 1948), 66; see also Jules Michelet, *La Sorcerie* (Paris: Marcel Didier, 1952, 1st edn 1862), 144.

[31] Ewen, *Witchcraft*, 145; Rueff, *Expert Midwife*, 61.

[32] Anon., *Extraordinary Life and Character of Mary Bateman, the Yorkshire Witch* (Leeds: Baines, 1809), 12.

[33] Robert Latham and William Matthews (eds), *The Diary of Samuel Pepys* (London: Bell, 1971), V, 275. For similar abortionist activities in France in the 1660s see the letters of Guy Patin in Pierre Bayle, *Dictionnaire historique et critique* (Paris: Desoeur, 1820), II, 449–50.

[34] Pechey, *Compleat Midwife*, 346.

[35] Defoe, *Augusta Triumphans*, 9; Daniel Defoe, *Moll Flanders* (Cambridge, Mass.: Riverside Press, 1959), 146–7.

[36] F. Grose, *Guide to Health, Beauty, Riches, and Honour* (London: Hooper, 1783), 12. A small book of 1752 referred to women 'repairing to persons of their own sex who live about Ludgate Hill and St Martin's Lane and put out handbills for the cure of all disorders to women'. Anon., *Low Life* (London, 1764 edn), 88–9. It could be that this work was the basis for a later claim that quacks 'cause hand-bills to be delivered to women, to acquaint them where they may apply for a medicine, that will inevitably cause an abortion'. Anon., *Essay on Quackery, and the Dreadful Consequences Arising from taking Advertised Medicines* (Kingston upon Hull: Clayton, 1805), 112.

[37] William Buchan, *Domestic Medicine or, the Family Physician* (London: Kelly, 1827), xiii.

[38] Quaife, *Wanton Wenches*, 119.

[39] Garth, *Dispensary*, IX, 434.

[40] Randolph Trumbach, *The Rise of the Egalitarian Family: Aristocratic kinship and domestic relationships in eighteenth-century England* (New York: Academic, 1978), 171.

[41] Spenser, *The Faerie Queene*, III (ii), 50.

[42] Enid Porter, *Cambridgeshire Customs and Folklore* (New York: Barnes & Noble, 1969), 10–11; John Gerarde, *The Herbal or General Historie of Plants* (London: Norton, 1636), 60; John Swan, *Speculum Mundi, or a Glasse Representing the Face of the World* (Cambridge: Buck & Daniel, 1635), 262.

[43] Leonard Sowerby, *The Ladies Dispensatory* (London: Ibbotson, 1651), 158–61; and see also Sir Thomas Browne, *Common Errors* in *Works*, ed. S. Wilkins (London: Pickering, 1835), III, 183.

[44] Quaife, *Wanton Wenches*, 120.

[45] Philip Barrough, *The Method of Physick* (London: Vautroullier, 1583), 147; R. Bunworth, *The Doctoresse* (London: Bourne, 1656), 10; James Primerose, *Popular Errours, or the Errours of the People in Physick* (London: Wilson, 1651), 305.

[46] Rueff, *Expert Midwife*, 60.

[47] Beryl Rowland (ed.), *The Medieval Woman's Guide to Health: The first English gynaecological handbook* (London: Croom Helm, 1981), 97.

[48] William Langham, *The Garden of Health* (London, 1578), 4, 254, 555; Gerarde, *Herbal*, 60.

[49] Sowerby, *Dispensatory* 158–61; see also William Williams, *Occult Physicke* (London: Leach, 1660), 94.

[50] See S. Chandrasekhar, *Abortion in a Crowded World: The problem of abortion with special reference to India* (London: Allen & Unwin, 1974), 54.

[51] A. Taussig, *Abortion, Spontaneous and Induced* (London: Kimpton, 1936); B.E., *A New Canting Dictionary of the Terms Ancient and Modern of the Canting Crew* (London, 1699); F. Grose, *A Classical Dictionary of the Vulgar Tongue* (London, S. Hooper, 1785). 'Poisoned' was still used to mean pregnant by the nineteenth-century author of *My Secret Life*; see G. Legnum, *Rationale of the Dirty Joke* (New York: Grove, 1968), 423.

[52] Eugene B. Brody, *Sex, Contraception, and Motherhood in Jamaica* (Cambridge, Mass.: Harvard University Press, 1981), 45.

[53] See the Wellcome Institute for the History of Medicine's collection of unpublished receipt books: Ann Brumwich MS 160; Lady Sleigh MS 751; Lady Miller MS 3547; Johanna St John MS 4338; Miss Frances Springatt MS 4683; Letitia Owen MS 3730; Abigail Smith MS 4631; Mrs Finger MS 2363.

[54] Jehan Goeuriot, *The Regiment of Life*, tr. Thomas Phayre (London, 1544), fol. lviii.

[55] Andrew Boorde, *The Breviary of Helthe* (London, 1547), lxxxiii; and see also John XXI, *The Treasuri of Helth*, tr. Humfre Lloyd (London: Coplande, 1558), xlvi; Langham, *Garden*, 4, 254, 477, 547, 555; Thomas Newton, *Approved Medicine and Cordial Receipts* (London: Marshe, 1580), 26–42; Sir Kenelm Digby, *Choice and Experiemental Receipts in Physicke and Chirgery* (London: Brome, 1675), 35; Peter Levens, *A Right Profitable Booke for all Diseases* (London: White, 1582), 104; John Freind, *Emmenologia* (London: Cox, 1729).

[56] Elizabeth Smith, *The Compleat Houswife* (London, 1725), 237, 320, 324; and see also Catharine Brooks, *The Compleat English Cook* (London: Cook, 1765), 120–1; Hannah Wooley, *The Accomplisht Ladys Delight* (London: Harris, 1677), 152.

[57] John Gregory, *Medical Lectures* (London, n.p., 1770), 379; Henry Manning, *A Treatise on Female Diseases* (London: Baldwin, 1775), 63–82; John Wesley, *Primitive Physicke* (London: Hawes, 1776), 90.

[58] A. Hume, *Every Woman Her Own Physician or, the Lady's Medical Assistant* (London, 1776), 16; John Aikin, *A Manual of Materia Medica* (Yarmouth: Downes & March, 1785), *passim*.

[59] Anon., *Complete Herbal or Family Physician* (London, 1787), I, 28, 234, 283, II, 33, 103; *Nicholas Culpeper's English Physician and Complete Herbal* (London, 1798), I, 340.

[60] James Primerose, *Popular Errours, or the Errours of the People in Physicke* (London, 1651), 305, 309; John Sadler, *The Sick Woman's Private Looking Glass* (Norwood, N.J.: W. J. Johnson, 1977, first edn 1656), 142 and see also Nicholas Culpeper, *A Directory for Midwives* (London: Cole, 1656), 70.

[61] Robert Christison, *A Treatise on Poisons* (Edinburgh: Black, 1829), 670–1; *Lancet*, I (1829–30), 74, 168–9; Richard Carlile, *Every Woman's Book* (London: Carlile, 1838), 23–4.

[62] Robert T. Gunther (ed.), *The Greek Herbal of Dioscorides* (Oxford: Oxford University Press, 1934), 270; *The Compleat Herbal or, Family Physician* (Manchester: Swindalls, 1787), II, 33; Robert Pemell, *The Second Part of the Treatise . . . of Physical Simples* (London: Legatt, 1653); Anon., *The Express: or Every Man His Own Doctor* (Gainsborough: Arundel, 1823).

[63] *Folklore*, 40 (1929), 118.

[64] Anon., *A Dictionary of English Plantnames* (London: Trubner, 1886), 416.

[65] Summers, *Malleus*, 66; see also Rowland, *Medieval Woman*, 135.

[66] F. G. Emmison, *Elizabethan Life: Morals and the Church courts* (Chelmsford: Essex County Council, 1973), 41–2; and see also Peter Treveris, tr. Anon., *The Grete Herbal* (London, 1526), cccc; William Turner, *The First and Second Parts of the Herbal* (London: Birckman, 1568).

[67] A. D. J. Macfarlane, 'The regulation of maternal and sexual relationships in seventeenth-century England, with special reference to the County of Essex' (London School of Economics, unpublished, M.Phil. thesis 1968), 154.

[68] William Coles, *Adam in Eden, or Natures Paradise* (London: John Streater, 1657), 593; see also John Archer, *A Compendious Herbal* (London, 1673), 129; Robert Lovell, *A Compleat Herbal* (Oxford: Davies, 1665), 385; Tryon, *An English Herbal* (London: A.C., 1726), 55.

[69] Anon., *Compleat Herbal*, II, 103; William Meyrick, *The New Family Herbal* (Birmingham: Pearson, 1790), 412; and see also Joseph Miller, *Botanicum Officinale: or a Compendious Herbal* (London: Bell, 1722).

[70] Spenser, *The Faerie Queene*, III (ii), 49.

[71] Abraham Cowley, *Poetical Blossomes* (London, n.p., 1633), 52; Dryden, *Juvenal*, 195; Thomas Middleton, *A Game at Chess* (London: Benn, 1966), 17.

[72] Samuel Ashwell, *A Practical Treatise on the Diseases Peculiar to Women* (London: Highley, 1844), 81.

[73] See the advertisements for pills of savin and mugwort in 'A Physician' *The Ladies Physical Directory* (London: Gentlewoman's, 1727).

[74] A. C. Wootton, *Chronicles of Pharmacy* (London: Macmillan, 1910), II, 163–4; P. S. Brown, 'Medicines advertised in eighteenth-century Bath newspapers', *Medical History*, 20 (1976), 152–68 and 'Female pills and the reputation of iron as an abortifacient', *Medical History*, 21 (1977), 291–304.

[75] In the industrial districts even workers would have recourse to new manufactured pharmaceuticals: see William Buchan *et al.*, *The Cottage Physician and Family Advisor* (London: Sherwood, 1825), 59.

185

[76] Theophilus Redwood (ed.), *Gray's Supplement to the Pharmacopoeia* (London: Longman, 1847), 450, 501–2, 527–8, 593; Malcolm Potts, Peter Diggory and John Peel, *Abortion* (Cambridge: Cambridge University Press, 1977), ch. 5.

[77] Edward Shorter, *A History of Women's Bodies* (New York: Basic Books, 1982), 177–224.

[78] On herbal abortifacients used in other cultures see George Devereux, *A Study of Abortion in Primitive Societies* (London: Yoseloff, 1960); Judith Bolyard, *Medicinal Plants and Home Remedies of Appalachia* (Springfield, Illinois: 1981), 26, 33, 85, 94; Walter H. Lewis and M. P. F. Elvin-Lewis, *Medical Botany* (London: John Wiley, 1977), 320–3; Lily M. Perry, *Medicinal Plants of East and South-East Asia* (Cambridge, Mass.: M.I.T. Press, 1980), *passim*; Malcolm Potts *et al.*, *Traditional Abortion Practices* (Triangle Park, N.C.: International Fertility Research Program, 1981).

[79] Enzo Nardi, *Procurato aborto del mondo greco-romano* (Milan: Guiffre, 1971).

[80] Devereux, *Abortion, passim*.

[81] Revd Thomas Oswald Cockayne, *Leechdoms, Wortcunning, and Starcraft of Early England*, ed. C. Singer (London: Holland Press, 1961), III, 147.

[82] John Wyclif, I Kings XVII, 22.

[83] Jehan Palsgrave, *Lesclairrcissement de la langue française* (London, 1530), 677–1.

[84] Thomas Wilson, *The Arte of Rhetorique* (London: n.p., 1553), 29.

[85] Christopher Hooke, *The Child-birth or Woman's Lecture* (London: Orwin, 1590), B.

[86] Lord Bryskett, *A Discourse on Civil Life* (London: Aspley, 1606), 44; and see also *Les Admirables secrets d'Albert le Grand* (Cologne, n.p., 1722), 10.

[87] Stephen Blancard, *Physical Dictionary* (London: Crouch, 1702), 48; cf. 140.

[88] James Guillemeau, *Child Birth* (London: Hatfield, 1612), 69–70.

[89] John Maubray, *The Female Physician, Containing all the Diseases Incident to that Sex* (London: Holland, 1724), 24–8.

[90] *Aristotle's Masterpiece: or, Secrets of Generation* (London: Howe, 1690), 13; A Physician [Nicolas Venette], *Conjugal Love Reveal'd* (London: Hinton, 1720), 62; and see also Sadler, *Sick Woman*, 142; William Sermon, *The Ladies Companion, or the English Midwife* (London: Edward Thomas, 1671), 23; R.C. *et al.*, *The Compleat Midwife's Practice Enlarged* (London: Brook, 1663), 93; Pechey, *Midwife*, 299.

[91] Thomas Denman, *An Introduction to the Practice of Midwifery* (London: Cox, 7th edn 1832).

[92] Daniel Blake Smith, *Inside the Great House: Planter family life in eighteenth-century Chesapeake society* (Ithaca, N.Y.: Cornell University Press, 1980), 28.

⁹³ William Shakespeare, *Othello*, IV, ii; John Ray, *The Wisdom of God Manifested in the Works of Creation* (London, 1691), 74; Richard Blackmore, *Prince Arthur* (London: Scolar Press, 1971 (1st edn 1695)), II, 26; Thomas Urquhart, *The First (Second) Book of Mr Francis Rabelais* (London, n.p., 1653).

⁹⁴ Procopius, tr. H. B. Dewing, *The Anecdota or Secret History* (Cambridge, Mass: Harvard University Press, 1935), VI, 203.

⁹⁵ Latham, *Pepys*, IV, 1.

⁹⁶ The eighteenth century witnessed the emergence of a utilitarianist logic that could be employed to defend abortion from a more modern philosophical position. For example, Locke's assault on the concept of innate ideas led him to imply that until birth a foetus could be said to have neither a soul nor a mind. 'He, I say, who considers this will perhaps find reason to imagine a *foetus* in the *mother's womb differs not much from the state of a vegetable*, but passes the greater part of its time without perception or thought, doing very little but sleep. . . .' John Locke, *An Essay Concerning Human Understanding* (1690: new edn New York: Dutton, 1961), I, 88. See the response of Thomas Beconsall that only 'monsters' destroyed their young; *Foundations of Natural Religion* (London: Rogers, 1698), 127–8. William Rowley agreed with Locke that the foetus had no soul until it breathed: *The Rational Practice of Physic* (London: Newberry, 1793), II, 41. Jeremy Bentham followed the argument that sensations were required to create ideas in attacking the laws on abortion and infanticide: *The Theory of Legislation*, ed. C. K. Ogden (London: Routledge & Kegan Paul, 1931), 264–5; 479–94. William Godwin was even more daring. In *Thoughts Occasioned by the Perusal of Dr Parr's Spital Sermon* (London: Taylor & Wilks, 1801), 65–6, he declared: 'Neither do I regard a new born child with any superstitious reverence. If the alternative were complete, I had rather such a child should perish in the first hour of its existence, than that a man should spend seventy years in a state of misery and vice.' And turning from the subject of infanticide to that of abortion he went on to report, 'In the island of Ceylon, for example, it appears to be a part of the common law of the country, that no woman shall be a mother before she is thirty, and they accordingly have their methods for procuring abortions, which we are told, are perfectly innoxious.' Godwin's purpose in drawing such information to his readers' attention was to show that before judging any act a comprehensive view had to be taken of its consequences. Both abortion and infanticide could be considered beneficial to the community if the pain they entailed was more than offset by avoidance of vice and misery. Such arguments were to have little impact on popular opinions and are only noted here because they foreshadowed the line of attack taken up by abortion reformers in the late nineteenth century. In the eighteenth century the discussion of abortion remained focused on the traditional right of the woman, before quickening, to take whatever measures she thought necessary. For responses to Godwin see John Bowles, *Reflections on the Political*

and Moral State of Society at the Close of the Eighteenth Century (London: Rivington, 1802), 134, and the slurs of Isaac Disraeli in Flim Flams cited in R. G. Grylls, William Godwin and His World (London: Oldhams, 1953), 159.

[97] K. Cangiamila, Abrégé de l'embryologie sacrée (Paris: n.p., 1745, 2nd edn 1762), 11–12, cf. 30.

[98] M. Des-Essartz, Traité de l'éducation corporelle (Paris, n.p., 1760), 18. Pierre Bayle noted that even priests used the term 'abortion' only to refer to the miscarriages of women who had already quickened and not to those who 'took early precautions and before the ensoulment took place'. Bayle, Dictionnaire, 452.

[99] Defoe, Conjugal Lewdness, 152.

[100] Some indication of the incidence of abortion at the end of the period is contained in an 1818 report on 400 women's childbearing histories. 128 had miscarried at least once and altogether had 305 miscarriages of which one half were 'constitutional' and one half 'accidental'. The investigator found that the consequences were not as serious as feared: 'by far the greatest number of miscarriages have occurred, alternatively, with pregnancies conducted to their full and happy termination'. This suggests that some at least were induced as a means of spacing births. See A. B. Granville, A Report of the Practice of Midwifery at the Westminster General Dispensary During 1818 (London: Burgess & Hill, 1819), 40, 42, 52.

[101] Boorde, Breviary, Fol. ix.

[102] Henry Bracken, The Midwife's Companion (London: Clarke, 1737), 84.

5 'Converting this measure of security into a crime'

[1] The law on abortion appears somewhat similar to the eighteenth-century Black Act inasmuch as both implied a growing impersonality of relations and the ruling classes' perceived need for law to replace moral coercion. See E. P. Thompson, Whigs and Hunters: The origin of the Black Act (London: Allen Lane, 1975).

[2] John T. Noonan et al., The Morality of Abortion (Cambridge, Mass.: Harvard University Press, 1970).

[3] Glanville Williams, The Sanctity of Life and the Criminal Law (London: Faber & Faber, 1958), 178.

[4] Joseph Bingham, Origines Ecclesiasticae: or, The Antiquities of the Christian Church (London: Straker, 1843), 210.

[5] Bingham, Origines, 211.

[6] See B. D. H. Miller, 'She who hath drunk any potion', Medium Aevum, 31 (1962), 188–93.

[7] Frederick J. Furnivall (ed.), Robert of Brunne's 'Handlying Synne' (A.D. 1303) (London: Kegan Paul, 1901), ll. 8333–42.

[8] Geoffrey Chaucer, *Canterbury Tales* (New York: Houghton-Mifflin, 1933; London: Macmillan, 1974), 292.

[9] Thomas Wilson, *The Arte of Rhetorique* (London, 1553), f. 29.

[10] Cited in Richard L. Greaves, *Society and Religion in Elizabethan England* (Minneapolis: University of Minnesota Press, 1981), 237.

[11] Noonan, *Abortion*, 27.

[12] Noonan, *Abortion*, 34.

[13] William Gouge, *Of Domesticall Duties* (London: Miller, 1634) and see also Jean Calvin, *Opera* (Brunsvigae: Berolini, 1863–1900), XXIV, 625; Richard Baxter, *A Christian Directory* (London: n.p., 1673), IV, 52.

[14] John Weemse, *An Exposition of the Moral Laws* in *Works* (London: Bellamie, 1636), 87, 98; see also John Donne, *Sermons*, ed. E. M. Simpson (Berkeley: University of California Press, 1953), VI, 270.

[15] Weemse, *Exposition*, 96–7.

[16] Cited in John T. McNeil and Helena M. Ganer, *Medieval Handbooks of Penance* (New York: Columbia University Press, 1938), 166, 197.

[17] On the courts see Anon., *The Ecclesiastical Courts* (London: SPCK, 1954); F. G. Emmisson, *Elizabethan Life: Morals and the Church Courts* (Chelmsford: Essex County Council, 1973); Brian L. Woodcock, *Medieval Ecclesiastical Courts in the Diocese of Canterbury* (Oxford: Oxford University Press, 1952); Revd J. S. Purvis, *An Introduction to Ecclesiastical Records* (London: St Antony's Press, 1953).

[18] Ralph Houlbrooke, *Church Courts and the People* (Oxford: Oxford University Press, 1975), 78.

[19] Paul Hair, *Before the Bawdy Courts* (New York: Barnes & Noble, 1972), 81, 152, 172, 204.

[20] On the avoidance of scandal see Keith Wrightson, 'Two concepts of order: justices, constables and jurymen in seventeenth-century England', in John Brewer and John Sayles (eds), *An Ungovernable People: The English and their Law in the Seventeenth and Eighteenth Centuries* (London: Hutchinson, 1980), 25–46; Caroline Bingham, 'Seventeenth-century attitudes towards deviant sex', *Journal of Interdisciplinary History*, 1 (1971), 465. Ralph Houlbrooke, Richard Helmholz and Geoffrey Quaife very kindly enlightened me on the workings of the ecclesiastical courts.

[21] But for the continued use of moral coercion against abortion see Harold W. Brace (ed.), *The First Minute Book of the Gainsborough Monthly Meeting of the Society of Friends* (Lincoln Record Society, 1949), II, 116.

[22] Christopher Hill, 'The Bawdy Courts', *Society and Puritanism in Pre-Revolutionary England* (London: Secker & Warburg, 1964), 305–7.

[23] Donald Veall, *The Popular Movement for Law Reform, 1640–1660* (Oxford: Clarendon, 1970), 139.

[24] For some interesting insights into the relationship of law and morality from the seventeenth century onwards see Ronald Hamowy, 'Medicine and the criminalization of sin: "Self-abuse in nineteenth-

century America"', *Journal of Libertarian Studies*, 1 (1977), 230.

[25] G. E. Woodbine (ed.), *Bracton on the Laws and Customs of England* (Cambridge, Mass.: Harvard University Press, 1968), 341.

[26] H. G. Richardson (ed.), *Fleta* (London: Seldon Society, 1955), LXXII, 60–1.

[27] Edward Coke, *The Third Part of the Institutes of the Laws of England* (London: Flesher, 1644), 50; see also William Hawkins, *A Treatise of the Pleas of the Crown* (London: Sayer, 1724), XXXI, Sect. 16.

[28] Matthew Hale, *Pleas of the Crown* (London: R. Atkyns, 1682), 53.

[29] Hale, *Pleas*, 126.

[30] William Blackstone, *Commentaries on the Laws of England* (London: n.p., 1765), I, 129.

[31] *The Laws Respecting Women* (London: J. Johnson, 1777), 348.

[32] It is significant that abortion is not even mentioned in William Eden's *Principles of Penal Law* (London: White, 1771).

[33] Bernard M. Dickens states that cases of abortion coming to court were rare in the eighteenth century: 'references to the procuring of abortion as a crime at common law before it became a statutory offence in 1803 are not numerous, and are fairly late in date'. *Abortion and the Law* (London: MacGibbon & Kee, 1966), 23. John Beattie has informed me that he did not come across any references to abortion in the quarter sessions or assizes of the counties he looked at between 1660 and 1800.

[34] See for example M. C. Versluysen, 'Lying-in hospitals in eighteenth-century London', in Helen Roberts (ed.), *Women, Health and Reproduction* (London: Routledge & Kegan Paul, 1981), 3–49; Jeanne Donnison, *Midwives and Medical Men: A history of inter-professional rivalries and women's rights* (London: Heinemann, 1977).

[35] John Hull (ed.), J. L. Baudelocque, *Two Memoirs on the Caesarian Operation* (Manchester: Sowler & Russell, 1801), 200.

[36] See Dorothy McLaren, 'Fertility, infant mortality, and breast feeding in the eighteenth century', *Medical History*, 22 (1978), 378–96; and 'Nature's contraceptive: wet-nursing and prolonged lactation: the case of Chesham, Buckinghamshire, 1578–1601', *Medical History*, 22 (1978), 378–96; 23 (1979), 426–41.

[37] Hull, *Caesarian*, 202.

[38] Thomas Denman, *An Introduction to the Practice of Midwifery* (London: Cox, 7th edn 1832) 333. On factory work and difficult births see also the statements made by Thomas Young, a Bolton physician, and Sir William Blizzard, a London surgeon, to the Committee on Child Labour in *Parliamentary Papers*, 15 (1831–2), 10610, 11222.

[39] Thomas Radford, *Observations on the Caesarian Section, Craniotomy, and Other Obstetric Operations* (London: Churchill, 1880).

[40] The first successful Caesarian in Britain was actually carried out in 1738 by an illiterate Irish midwife equipped only with a razor. John Burton (satirized as Dr Slop by Sterne in *Tristram Shandy*) was the first doctor to defend the operation in England; see his *An Essay Towards a*

Complete New System of Midwifery (London: Hodges, 1751). Interest was also expressed by John Aitken, *Principles of Midwifery* (Edinburgh, 1785). For overviews see J. Paul Pundel, *Histoire de l'opération césarienne* (Brussels: Presses académiques européennes, 1969) and J. H. Young, *Caesarian Section: The history and development of the operation from earliest times* (London: Lewis, 1944).

41 Harvey Graham, *Eternal Eve: The mysteries of birth and the customs that surround it* (London: Hutchinson, 1960), 200.

42 William Simmons, *Reflections on the Propriety of Performing the Caesarian Operation* (Manchester: Clarkes, 1798); John Hull, *A Defence of the Caesarian Operation* (Manchester: Bickerstaff, 1798); John Simmons, *A Detection of the Fallacy of Dr. Hull's Defence of the Caesarian Operation* (Manchester: Sowler & Russell, 1798); John Hull, *Observations on Mr. Simmons' Detections* (Manchester: Bickerstaff, 1799).

43 On induction see Samuel Merriman, *A Synopsis of the Various Kinds of Difficult Parturition* (London: Callow, 1814), 179; Denman, *Introduction*, 321; Robert Barnes, 'On the indications and operations for the induction of premature labour and for the acceleration of labour', *Obstetrical Society of London: Transactions*, III (1861), 107–41; W. Bathurst Woodman and C. Meymott Tidy, *A Handy Book of Forensic Medicine* (London, n.p., 1877), 745; J. Munro et al., *Historical Review of British Obstetrics and Gynaecology, 1800–1950* (London: Livingston, 1950), 33–4. In France the Caesarian operation was not without its opponents. J. F. Sacombe formed an 'école anti-césarienne de Paris'. See his *Plus d'opération césarienne ou le voeu de l'humanité* (Paris: Peronneau, 1797).

44 John Burns, *The Principles of Midwifery* (London: Longman, 1837), 313.

45 It was asserted that craniotomy was six times more common in Britain than in France; see Fleetwood Churchill, *The Theory and Practice of Midwifery* (London: n.p., 1853). For later critiques of the process see W. O. Priestly and H. R. Storer (eds), *The Obstetric Memoirs and Contributions of J. Y. Simpson* (Edinburgh: J. C. Black, 1856), I, 506 ff., 656–62. Simpson asserted that both craniotomies and Caesarians could be avoided by version, the turning of the child, to permit normal delivery.

46 See for example Fielding Ould, *A Treatise of Midwifery* (London: Nelson, 1742), 143 ff.; William Dease, *Observations in Midwifery* (Dublin: Williams, 1783), 60 ff.; William Osborn, *An Essay on Laborious Parturition* (London: Cadell, 1783).

47 Osborn, *An Essay*, 64.

48 Cited in Simmons, *Reflections*, 27.

49 Simmons, *A Detection*, 89–90.

50 On French Catholic views see Phillipe Peu, *La pratique des acouchemens* (Paris, 1794); L'abbé Cangiamilia, *Abrégé de l'embryologée sacrée*, tr. père Dinouart (Paris: Nyon, 1775); Pierre Darmon, *Le mythe*

de la procréation à l'âge baroque (Paris: Pauvret, 1977), 230–1; Young, *Caesarian*, 39. Laurence Sterne provided his readers with a full account of the Sorbonne deliberations, which he in turn drew from Heinrich van Deventer, *Observations importantes sur le manuel des accouchemens* (1734). See Laurence Sterne, *Tristram Shandy*, ed. Howard Anderson (New York: Norton, 1980; Oxford: Oxford University Press, 1983), 44–5.

[51] Ould, *Midwifery*, 198; Merriman, *A Synopsis*, 171; J. Blondel, *Principles and Practices of Obstetrics* (London: Butler, 1840); F. Ramsbotham, *The Principles and Practices of Obstetrical Medicine and Surgery* (London: Churchill, 1844).

[52] Denman, *Introduction* (1794 edn), II, 175, 172.

[53] Denman, *Introduction* (1832 edn), 332.

[54] Radford, *Observations*, 49.

[55] M. Pierce Rucker and Edwin M. Rucker, 'A librarian looks at Caesarian section', *Bulletin of the History of Medicine*, 25 (1951), 137.

[56] Denman, *Introduction* (1794), II, 172.

[57] Samuel Farr, *Elements of Medical Jurisprudence* (London, 1788), 41.

[58] Denman, *Introduction* (1832), 322.

[59] Merriman, *Synopsis*, 181.

[60] Leon Radzinowicz, *A History of English Criminal Law and its Administration from 1750* (London: Stevens, 1948), I; William C. Townsend, *The Lives of Twelve Eminent Judges* (London: Longman, 1846), 324–38; *Hansard*, 36 (March 28 1803), 1246–7.

[61] Barbara A. Hanawalt, *Crime and Conflict in English Communities, 1300–1348* (Cambridge, Mass.: Harvard University Press, 1979), 154–6; R. H. Helmholz, 'Infanticide in the province of Canterbury during the fifteenth century', *History of Childhood Quarterly*, 2 (1975), 379–90; Y.-B. Brissaud, 'L'Infanticide à la fin du moyen âge', *Revue historique de droit français et étranger*, 50 (1972), 229–56.

[62] Joan Kent, 'Attitudes of Members of the House of Commons to the regulation of "Personal Conduct" in late Elizabethan and early Stuart England', *Bulletin of the Institute for Historical Research*, 46 (1973), 41–52.

[63] Peter C. Hoffer and N. E. H. Hull, *Murdering Mothers: Infanticide in England and New England, 1558–1803* (New York: New York University Press, 1981); Keith Wrightson, 'Infanticide in earlier seventeenth-century England', *Local Population Studies*, 15 (1975), 19–22; Thomas R. Forbes, ' "By what disease or casualty": the changing face of death in London', *Journal of the History of Medicine and Allied Sciences*, 31 (1976), 415; P. E. H. Hair, 'Deaths from violence in Britain: a tentative secular survey', *Population Studies*, 25 (1971), 5–25.

[64] Cited in Hoffer and Hull, *Mothers*, 20.

[65] Alan Macfarlane, 'Illegitimacy and illegitimates in English history', in P. Laslett *et al.*, *Bastardy and its Comparative History* (London: Edward Arnold, 1980), 71–86.

[66] R. W. Malcolmson, 'Infanticide in the eighteenth century', in J. S. Cockburn (ed.), *Crime in England, 1500–1800* (London: Methuen, 1977); J. M. Beattie, 'The criminality of women in eighteenth-century England', *Journal of Social History*, 8 (1974–5), 84–5.

[67] See for example the case of a woman who strangled her child but was acquitted in October of 1733 because the infant resulted from an incestuous relationship; also the case of a servant who hid her dead baby's body in a wig box and was acquitted in June of 1734 because of her possession of an infant's shirt, cap and stay: *The Proceedings at the Sessions of the Peace . . . for the City of London and County of Middlesex* (London: Wilford, 1737), 10, 136.

[68] Anon., *A Rebuke to the Sin of Uncleanness* (London: Downing, 1704), 6; William Walsh, 'A dialogue concerning women,' in *Works* (London: E. Curll, 1736), 156; and see also John Scott, *The Fatal Consequences of Licentiousness: A sermon* (Hull: Ferraby, 1810).

[69] Robert Burton, *The Anatomy of Melancholy* (London: n.p., 1621, 2nd edn 1632), 159–60.

[70] A. Clark (ed.), *The Life and Times of Anthony Wood* (Oxford: Oxford University Press, 1891–5), I, 250–1.

[71] Bernard de Mandeville, *A Modest Defense of the Public Stewes* (London: A. Moore, 1724), 4.

[72] Blackstone, *Commentaries*, I, 128; and see also Leon Radzinowicz, *A History of English Criminal Law* (London: Stevens), I, 432–6.

[73] *Parliamentary History of England*, 17 (1771–4), 452–3.

[74] Baron de Montesquieu, *The Spirit of the Laws*, ed. D. W. Carrithers (Berkeley: University of California Press, 1977), 26, ch. III, sect. 4; Cesare Beccaria, *On Crimes and Punishments* (New York: Bobbs-Merrill, 1963), 85–6.

[75] J. P. Brissot de Warville, *Les moyens d'adoucir la rigueur des loix penales en France* (Paris: n.p., 1780), 108.

[76] Jeremy Bentham, *The Theory of Legislation* (London: Routledge & Kegan Paul, 1931), 265.

[77] *Gentleman's Magazine*, 44 (1774), 462–3.

[78] William Cummin, *The Proofs of Infanticide Considered: Including Dr Hunter's tract on child murder* (London: Longman, 1836), 1–20; and see also William Hutchinson, *A Dissertation on Infanticide* (London: Sauter, 1821); James Simpson, *A Probationary Essay on Infanticide* (submitted to the Royal College of Surgeons of Edinburgh, 1825).

[79] *Hansard* (March 28, 1803), 1246.

[80] The Vagrant Act of 1810 (50 Geo. III c. 51) allowed justices to commit a 'lewd woman' with an illegitimate child to prison for twelve months and the Vagrant Act of 1824 (5 Geo. IV c. 83) allowed one month's imprisonment for 'Idle and disorderly persons' and three months for 'Rogues and vagabonds' who would include those who concealed a birth or abandoned a child. Married women were not prosecuted for concealment until the passage of the Offences Against

the Person Act of 1828 (9 Geo. IV c. 31). 9 Geo. IV c. 34 allowed a simple concealment charge to be filed; the 1803 statute assumed that the woman would first be tried for murder and then for concealment. In 1849 Rebecca Smith was the last woman in England to be executed for infanticide. See Hoffer and Hull, *Mothers*, 87; Nigel Walker, *Crime and Insanity in England* (Edinburgh: Edinburgh University Press, 1968), II, 126–8; J. W. Jeudine, *Observations on English Criminal Law and Procedure* (London: King, 1968), 126–8.

[81] *Parliamentary History of England*, 36 (1801–3), 1246; *Journal of the House of Lords*, 44 (1802–4), II, 265, 286; *Journal of the House of Commons*, 58 (1802–3), 425, 509, 514, 516. On developments elsewhere see L. Lewin, *Die Fruchtabtreibung durch Gifte und andere Mittel* (Berlin: Springer, 1922).

[82] Bentham, *Legislation*, 493–4. These unpublished statements were written in the period 1814–16. For similar sentiments see the letter of Francis Place to Richard Carlile (17 August 1822, Place Papers, British Museum), 68 (89).

[83] James Fitzjames Stephen, *History of the Criminal Law of England* (London: Macmillan, 1883), III, 116.

[84] Alexander Burnett, *The Medical Advertiser* (London: Lacey & Knight, 1824), 293.

[85] Sir Edmund Head, *Report on the Law of Bastardy, With a Supplementary Report on a Cheap Remedy for Seduction* (London: Clowes, 1840). Head's argument is suspect, however, inasmuch as it complemented his campaign against the laws on affiliation. He asserted that if such laws were retained the result would be for seducers to force their victims to have recourse to abortion.

[86] *Legal Examiner*, II (17 March–1 September 1832), 36. See also George Greaves, 'Observations on some causes of infanticide', *Transactions of the Manchester Statistical Society* (1863–4), 19–41.

[87] O. W. Bartley, *A Treatise on Forensic Medicine* (London: Barry, 1815), 2.

[88] William Buchan, *Domestic Medicine* (Leith: Allardice, 1816), 403.

[89] Dr Hutchinson, 'Medical jurisprudence', *London Medical and Physical Journal* (January, 1820), 97.

[90] John Burns, *Observations on Abortion* (London: Longman, 1806), 66.

[91] *Lancet*, 2 (1828–9), 54–5.

[92] Michael Ryan, *A Manual of Midwifery* (London: Renshaw & Rush: 1831), 206.

[93] Buchan, *Domestic Medicine*, 403. It is interesting to note that though the 1774 edition of *Domestic Medicine* states that abortion is dangerous it does not refer to it as a crime.

[94] John Gordon Smith, *The Principles of Forensic Medicine* (London: Underwood, 1821), 290.

[95] Thomas Radford, *The Value of the Embryonic and Foetal Life*,

Legally, Socially, and Obstetrically Considered (Manchester, n.p., 1848), 11.

⁹⁶ On doctors' difficulty in determining if women were pregnant see James Blundell, *Observations of Some of the More Important Diseases of Women* (London: Cox, 1837), 236 ff.; Alexander Hamilton, *A Treatise on Midwifery* (London: J. Murray, 1781), 160.

⁹⁷ Burns, *Observations*, 84.

⁹⁸ Bartley, *A Treatise*, 5.

⁹⁹ George Edward Male, *An Epitome of Juridical or Forensic Medicine* (London: Underwood, 1816), 206.

¹⁰⁰ Hutchinson, 'Medical jurisprudence', 13.

¹⁰¹ Smith, *Principles*, 294; J. A. Paris and J. S. M. Fonblanque, *Medical Jurisprudence* (London: Phillips, 1823), 89 ff.

¹⁰² T. R. Beck and W. Dunlop, *Elements of Medical Jurisprudence* (London: Anderson, 1825), 138.

¹⁰³ Beck and Dunlop, *Elements*, 140.

¹⁰⁴ Charles Severn, *First Lines of the Practice of Midwifery* (London: Highley, 1831), 134.

¹⁰⁵ Ryan, *Midwifery*, 205 and see also Michael Ryan, *A Manual of Medical Jurisprudence* (Edinburgh: Black, 1836), 28.

¹⁰⁶ Thomas Stewart Traill, *Outlines of a Course on Medical Jurisprudence* (Edinburgh: Black, 1836), 28.

¹⁰⁷ Dr A. T. Thompson, *Lancet* (28 June 1837), 626; and see also *London Medical and Chirurgical Journal*, n.s. 10 (1836–7), 882.

¹⁰⁸ B. T. Davis, 'George Edward Male, MD: The Father of English medical jurisprudence', *Proceedings of the Royal Society of Medicine*, 67 (1974), 117–200, provides an introductory overview of the subject. We have cited above the comments on abortion made in the forensic texts of Farr (1788), Dease (1793), Bartley (1815), Male (1816), Paris and Fonblanque (1825) and Bell and Dunlop (1825). Concern for abortion was also expressed in Andrew Duncan, *Heads of Lectures on Medical Police* (Edinburgh: Neill, 1801); J. W. Willcock, *The Laws Relating to the Medical Profession* (London: Strahan, 1830); J. Chitty, *A Practical Treatise on Medical Jurisprudence* (London: Longman, 1834).

¹⁰⁹ W. Ogilvie Porter, *Medical Science and Ethics* (Bristol: Strong, 1837), 27.

¹¹⁰ *The Trial of Charles Angus, Esq. on an Indictment for the Wilful Murder of Margaret Burns* (Liverpool: Jones, 1808) and see also Thomas R. Forbes, 'Early forensic medicine in England: the Angus murder trial', *Journal of the History of Medicine and Allied Sciences*, 37 (1981), 296–310.

¹¹¹ See James Gerard, *Vindications of the Opinions Delivered in Evidence by the Medical Witnesses for the Crown on a Late Trial at Lancaster for Murder* (Liverpool: Jones, 1808); James Carson, *Remarks on a Late Publication entitled 'A Vindication . . .'* (Liverpool: Jones, 1808; M. Royston, 'Historical sketch of the progress of medicine in the year

1809'; *Medical and Physical Journal*, 24 (July 1810), 38; James Dawson, *An Exposure of Some False Statements Contained in Dr Carson's Pamphlet* (Liverpool: Jones, 1809); D. Campbell, *Reflections Occasioned by the Perusal of a Pamphlet* (Liverpool: Jones, 1809); Paris and Fonblanque, *Jurisprudence*, II, 176; Thompson, *Lancet*, I (1836–7), 627. In Rex vs. Phillips (1812) doctors disagreed when a foetus could be said to quicken and the court declared that when a mother felt it move it was quick.

[112] Percival originally drew up the work as *Medical Jurisprudence, or a Code of Ethics and Institutes Adopted for the Profession of Physic and Surgery* in 1794; it was published as *Medical Ethics* (Manchester: J. Johnson, 1803).

[113] See for example Abraham Banks, *Medical Etiquette* (London: Fox, 1839).

[114] Ivan Waddington, 'The development of medical ethics: a socio-logical analysis', *Medical History*, 19 (1975), 38–51.

[115] On reform of the law see *Parliamentary Papers* VIII (1819), 42–3; *Parliamentary Papers*, II (1828), 333, 349, 365; *Parliamentary Papers*, II (1837), 709, 713. See also the Second Report of the Commissioners on Criminal Law in *Parliamentary Papers*, XXIV (1846), 147–8 in which it was suggested that the woman be held guilty of inducing her own miscarriage and that explicit provision be made for abortion 'done in good faith with the intention of saving the life of the woman'. The first recommendation was acted upon in the 1861 Offences Against the Person Act.

[116] Thomas Radford, *The Value of Embryonic and Foetal Life Legally, Socially, and Obstetrically Considered* (London, 1848), 4–7; Ryan, *Midwifery* (1841 edition), 163; Henry Bracken, *The Midwife's Companion* (London: J. Clarke, 1737), 36.

[117] On the later development of the abortion debate in America and Britain see James C. Mohr, *Abortion in America: The Origins and Evolution of National Policy, 1800–1900* (New York: Oxford University Press, 1978); R. Sauer, 'Infanticide and abortion in nineteenth-century Britain', *Population Studies*, 32 (1978), 81–94.

[118] Although it did not seem to play any role in the debate over abortion it is worth noting that English courts had declared from the mid-eighteenth century that in order to simplify inheritance cases a foetus was to be considered a living child. Ignoring the embryological and theological wrangles judges simply ruled that any child born within nine months of a parent's death to have full testamentary rights. Sir John Leach asserted in 1823:

> It is now fully settled that a child *en ventre sa mere* is within the intention of a gift to children *living* at the death of a testator; not because such a child (and especially in the early stages of conception) can strictly be considered as answering the description of a child

living; but because the potential existence of such a child places it plainly within the reason and motive of the gift.

Trower vs Butts, 1 Sim 7 Stu., 57 Eng Rep 72, 73 (Ch. 1823) and see also 2 Atk. 114, 117, 26 Eng Rep 472, 473 (Ch. 1740), Doe dem Clarke vs Clark, 2 HBL 399, 126 Eng Rep 617 (CP 1795), Thellusson vs Thellusson, 4 Ves. 227, 31 Eng Rep 117 (Ch. 1798).

[119] Jacques Donzelot, *The Policing of Families* (London: Hutchinson, 1980); Michel Foucault, *The History of Sexuality*, vol. 1: *An Introduction* (New York: Pantheon, 1978).

[120] Angus McLaren, *Birth Control in Nineteenth-Century England* (London: Croom Helm, 1978).

Conclusion

[1] W. A. Wright (ed.), *The Works of William Shakespeare* (London: Macmillan, 1866), 282.

[2] On the point that women in Africa sometimes seek to space births, not necessarily to limit family size but perhaps even to achieve an ultimately larger, healthier family, see Jane T. Bertrand, W. E. Bertrand and Miatudila Malonga, 'The use of traditional and modern methods of fertility control in Kinshasa, Zaire', *Population Studies*, 37 (1983), 129–36. Such findings lend support to the notion that some early nineteenth-century feminists shied away from public defences of contraception because they saw the woman's concern as being to provide for her children rather than to limit their number. See Barbara Taylor, *Eve and the New Jerusalem: Socialism and Feminism in the Nineteenth Century* (London: Virago, 1983), 216.

[3] For the argument that women in Africa might also have been 'freer' before the intrusion of new élites and their moral codes see James M. Ault, Jr, 'Making "modern" marriage "traditional": state power and the regulation of marriage in colonial Zambia', *Theory and Society*, 12 (1983), 181–210.

[4] Franklin F. Mendels, 'Proto-industrialization: the first phase of the industrialization process', *Journal of Economic History*, 32 (1972), 241–61; Peter Kriedte, Hans Medick and Jurgen Schumbohm, *Industrialization Before Industrialization: Rural industry in the genesis of capitalism* (Cambridge: Cambridge University Press, 1981); Moni Nag, 'How modernization can also increase fertility', *Current Anthropology*, 21 (1980), 571–87.

Index